# Chinese Medicine and the Management of Hypermobile Ehlers-Danlos Syndrome

# Chinese Medicine and the Management of Hypermobile Ehlers-Danlos Syndrome

A GUIDE FOR PRACTITIONERS

**Paula Bruno, Ph.D., L.Ac.**

Foreword by John Largess

SINGING DRAGON

LONDON AND PHILADELPHIA

First published in Great Britain in 2023 by Singing Dragon,
an imprint of Jessica Kingsley Publishers
Part of John Murray Press

1



Disclaimer: The information contained in this book is not intended to replace the services of trained medical professionals or to be a substitute for medical advice. You are advised to consult a doctor on any matters relating to your health, and in particular on any matters that may require diagnosis or medical attention.

A CIP catalogue record for this title is available from the British Library and the Library of Congress

ISBN 978 1 83997 498 4
eISBN 978 1 83997 499 1

Printed and bound in Great Britain by CPI Group (UK) Ltd, Croydon CR0 4YY

Jessica Kingsley Publishers' policy is to use papers that are natural, renewable and recyclable products and made from wood grown in sustainable forests. The logging and manufacturing processes are expected to conform to the environmental regulations of the country of origin.

Singing Dragon
Carmelite House
50 Victoria Embankment
London EC4Y 0DZ

www.singingdragon.com

John Murray Press
Part of Hodder & Stoughton Limited
An Hachette UK Company

# Contents

# Author's Note and Acknowledgments

The author wishes to begin by thanking her editors, Claire, Rosa, and Bonnie whose careful reading helped to unify the manuscript.

The use of Chinese medical terms in English and pinyin throughout the text follows a pattern. Organs in Chinese medicine are capitalized; their use to communicate Western concepts is not (Lung vs. lung, for example). The same goes for terms that we would use in Chinese medicine such as our use of the word "Wind" vs. the air that blows leaves from trees ("wind"). Common terms that people in the profession all know and use (yin, yang, qi, gua sha, and the like) are written just as they are here (no italics, no special emphasis). When the author directly quotes a scholar who did write with diacritics, these are replicated as their original writer produced them, including the tone marks.

She is especially grateful to her dear friend, Ainge Lin, who is a native speaker of Mandarin and who so graciously read the bibliography for correct renderings of Chinese names. Any remaining errors are the author's own.

The bibliography for this book is extensive. Most of the in-text citations are not from biomedical sources. These are recorded in the bibliography at the end of the book in MLA format. The sources in the notes are mostly scientific papers that are accessible online. The author provided URLs for these papers in the notes and created a bibliography, in APA format, which is available at uk.singingdragon.com/catalogue/book/9781839974984.

# Foreword

The world we live in today, at least for so many of us of a certain income and class, seems to promise better physical and mental health than ever before in human history. Western medicine has never before purported to understand more about nutrition, biochemistry, cellular biology, and disease pathology. Never before has such a wide range of mass-produced drugs and treatments for an equally wide range of ailments been manufactured and made available so easily and to so many people. Research and studies abound, as do scholarly journals devoted to every branch of the human organism.

And beyond the borders of Western biomedicine, for most us who have easy internet access, an even wider range of health modalities and traditions is available for our consideration at the touch of a keyboard or the swipe of a finger. Whatever our health issues, we can turn to traditional herbs and medicines from Europe, India, Tibet, China, and the indigenous peoples of the Americas among others; or to movement modalities such as Feldenkrais, Alexander Technique, or qi gong; or maybe we opt for physical massage and palpation and body manipulation techniques of an almost limitless variety; or perhaps we choose even the mental rigors of meditation if not one of the almost staggering array of purely energetic healing techniques that can be explored online and in social media.

And yet...

Who among us would claim that our health, no matter what its present state, in this moment feels assured and completely under our control?

On the contrary, for those of us who experience so many of the common health challenges, and especially those of us who either live with hypermobile Ehlers-Danlos syndrome or who are on the hypermobility spectrum, it can feel as if, despite an overwhelming barrage of health information being thrown at us, no one speaking seems to actually know much of anything at all. Or at least not anything that helps us feel better in an appreciable way.

Without a specialist willing to read, research, consider, and then to winnow critically through it, all the vast information on health we have access to today is of little value to an actual patient. Without a certain amount of intense study, coupled with the activation of techniques in practice with actual patients, any conceptual knowledge remains, at the end of the day, merely theoretical and of little impact to you or to me who are suffering.

I myself as a patient have benefited tremendously from just such a scholarly practice by a dedicated specialist in the person of Paula Bruno, Ph.D., L.Ac. Dr. Bruno's focus on Chinese medicine as delivered in a contemporary context dominated by Western biomedical culture and her application of this focus to my own somatic challenges has not only transformed my own health, but also elevated my own general understanding of what human health can and should be.

As a full-time performing classical concert musician and a university professor teaching the viola to both grad students and undergraduates, the health of my tendons, ligaments, and connective tissue is essential to what I do daily in a deeper way than for most humans. The health and function of these tissues in my body is reflected not only in the smoothness of motion and pain-free functionality that we all would hope for in everyday life, but even more so in the sounds I produce in my chosen art medium and the control and nuance that I can (or cannot) bring to my listeners' experience when I play music. My tendons are my voice, in the same way that the physicality of the vocal cords embody the true voice of the opera singer. I can truly say that the changes and improvements I have experienced under Dr. Bruno's treatment over time are to me both physically palpable and aesthetically audible.

As with many people, my own personal health journey throughout the course of my life has been a variegated one, with many twists and turns, highs and lows, and elements of surprise regularly mixed in. Notwithstanding, I can say with confidence that over the past several years, through treatments developed with Dr. Bruno's unique comparatist's approach to Chinese medicine and Western biomedicine, and under her tutelage and attentive care, I have never felt healthier, been more resistant to ailments of all kinds, or felt more confident in my ability to maintain my own good health...

All of it seems truly miraculous, to be honest. But as if that were not enough, her scholarly and insightful attitudes have inspired me to understand Chinese medicine itself more deeply, and to appreciate how every aspect of my mental and physical health can find reference and support in its simultaneously ancient and modern context. This opening of my understanding has been invaluable to me both as a patient and as a human being trying his best to lead a long and healthy life.

In the end, every patient must create healing for themselves. We who suffer look for good, confident guidance to point the way forward, but we must ultimately walk this path ourselves. Knowledge and experience that we can implement is essential to us, but even more essential are the values of critical thinking and study that have yielded these pearls of knowledge to our guides. A practitioner's role is first to heal, and then to teach.

I hope that all the advice, experience, and knowledge put forth in this book will be of inestimable value to hEDS patients and the practitioners who treat them. But I hope even more fervently that the philosophies of learning and wellness that underly all of the suggestions presented here will inspire an active and critical engagement with health in all who read this book.

*John Largess*
*Assistant Professor of Practice, University of Texas at Austin*
*Violist, Miró String Quartet*

# Introduction

The Ehlers-Danlos syndromes are a collection of heritable connective tissue disorders that affect the body across a wide range of systems and primarily target the skin, the joints, and the blood vessels.

Or so prevailing narratives tell us.

Dry, factual outlines such as the one that opens this introduction are commonly employed to introduce EDS and they are, one could suppose, an example of the proverb about the journey of a thousand steps beginning with the first one. Containing this disorder via genotype offers hope in the form of diagnosis. In truth, the Ehlers-Danlos syndromes (note the plural) are a hydra. If there is a diagnosis, this does not herald the journey's end. Instead, another pilgrimage begins. The steps required to arrive at a coherent narrative about ways to live with this disorder and even thrive, regardless, become a winding road that is unique to each patient. The average length of time a sufferer will spend in search of a diagnosis is ten to twelve years.

If diagnosed, then what?

Though not altogether unusual, hypermobile Ehlers-Danlos syndrome (hEDS) is categorized as a rare disorder. It is an exceptional physician who recognizes its signs and who is able to correctly address the issues at hand. Siloed medical care means that this hypermobile hero or heroine sees multiple different providers, some of whom might not know or care to learn about EDS. The long-haul slog for meaningful support becomes exhausting, demoralizing, and potentially fruitless.

And what of people who do not find recourse within the confines of biomedicine?

Chinese medicine is a uniquely suitable response to the ever-shifting vagaries of complex diseases in general. In particular, Chinese medicine is particularly adept at responding to a disorder that is based on connective tissue and expressed with the variability of an endlessly shifting tai chi symbol. Yet we need to evaluate and reevaluate our knowledge of this medicine when working with heritable connective tissue disorders. The terminology and significance of syndrome and pattern, already translated from the original classical Chinese into a multitude of world languages, does not capture the Ehlers-Danlos syndromes. This condition as it presents in clinic is unique on a case-by-case basis, too. To work with Ehlers-Danlos patients is to answer an invitation to become an exceptionally flexible, knowledgeable, and committed practitioner.

We have all seen an EDS patient, whether we knew it at the time or not. When we treated someone with undue allergic reaction to virtually everything, we may have gotten deeper into the realm of mast cell activation syndrome (MCAS) than we might have realized. Some of us will read *Chinese Medicine and the Management of Hypermobile Ehlers-Danlos Syndrome* (hereafter *Chinese Medicine*) and experience a dawning self-awareness. It can be a revelation to find that one is adjacent to, if not a part of, the hypermobile community. Perhaps the newfound comprehension includes a broader reading of one's own long-standing patterns of food sensitivity or hyper-reaction to prescription medication. My expectation for this book is that we will learn about our patients, we will develop an expanded perspective on Chinese medicine, and possibly—even—we might learn about ourselves. A tall order, but I stand behind my words.

This is an extraordinarily complex subject—the Ehlers-Danlos syndromes and how we as practitioners of Chinese medicine might address them—and the information we have at present is constantly shifting due to changes in scientific knowledge in confrontation with the needs of people who live with this condition. Neither scientific research nor Western biomedicine has all the answers. Chinese medicine does not have a syndrome pattern for EDS but we most certainly are in possession of ways to understand it and methods to improve the lot of those who live with it. We need to know how and where to be aware of red flags. We need to understand the norm for each individual body. (There are a few general types, but truly? Each one is unique.) We need to know how to tread lightly and remain within our scope of practice according to our local laws. What we offer as practitioners of Chinese medicine in so doing is of inestimable value.

The intent of *Chinese Medicine* is not to offer a fixed recipe. Instead, I provide a substantive outline of EDS presentations and consider options regarding strategy. I then suggest a framework for clinicians so that we might address, from within our systematic body of knowledge, each of our unique cases (and each one is so different) in a safe, effective, and knowledgeable way. Though we do not diagnose EDS, we most certainly can correctly identify what is in front of us. Though there is no cure, there are certainly approaches that can ameliorate suffering and benefit the wellbeing of our patients. To do this requires a genuine understanding of the hypermobile patient not just within their own bodies but, also, as part of their larger contextual milieux.

Synthesizing the vast amount of information that we need in order to provide safe, effective treatment was a challenge. In part, what I share here is the fruit of my first decade of clinical experience. I, too, discovered my own self when I learned about EDS and I share some epiphanies herein. Another foundation of this volume is derived from my first career. Before I was a practitioner of Chinese medicine, I was a Spanish professor with a background in comparative literature. My area specialty was national trauma and how it filtered through literature and art. This background is akin to that of a medical historian. My identity as a multicultural, multilingual scholar is writ large across every page of *Chinese Medicine*. When I study Asian medical traditions and engage with patients in all of their complexities, I draw upon this background. However, like many of us who practice outside of China, I am not Asian. I do not speak Chinese, and I live and practice far, far from Beijing. I am of Mediterranean heritage. These factors are all aspects of the way my professional identity expresses itself in clinical encounters and of the way I present the material in the following pages of this book.

Being able to work with EDS patients requires substantial knowledge and considerable intellectual agility. I put *Chinese Medicine* together in the way I would if I were teaching a course on intercultural competency, medical history, and critical thought in a language not native to my students. Since this course is neither in Spanish nor in Italian, I have been a learner too. The structure of each chapter reflects this process. Each one begins and concludes with a shorter section designed to introduce and reintroduce significant themes. These include diagnosis, the subject of pain, how we might build our communication skills, and topics related to the status of Chinese medicine both within and outside of China. I rely on the scholarship of anthropologists, sociologists, historians, and the odd literary allusion based on my own background as a Spanish professor. I also illuminate these themes via extensive endnotes. The information in each chapter is considerable. Anyone who wishes to expand upon what is contained therein will discover enough material for a lifetime of investigation by following the breadcrumb trails provided by the endnotes.

Chapter by chapter, we build understanding and mastery of an incredibly complicated collection of disorders.

Chapter one begins with biomedicine. To do so in no way privileges the Occident. Instead, it is intended to summarize the key themes surrounding the Ehlers-Danlos syndromes in particular and connective tissue disorder in general that everyone (both clinician and patient) must know. The Ehlers-Danlos syndromes are a biomedically defined entity and it wastes time to begin otherwise. There is a staggering amount of information available for clinicians and by summarizing as I have done, my aim is also to save readers quite a bit of energy. The areas that I underscore in the initial section represent common issues that I have seen in my clinic. I introduce red flags that might appear in the treatment rooms when we work with heritable connective tissue disorder (HCTD). With this outline in hand, a practitioner can follow up on the information contained in the main body of the text via the notes. With this resource, a practitioner saves time and mental energy.

This is also a matter of safety. There is a vast range of presentations intrinsic to this condition. A clinician who works with HCTDs will become familiar with the different potential norms for patients and, as I explain, it is incumbent upon us to listen to our patients and to step forward to reach them where they are, no matter what this might mean. (Given the variation in one's patients, this could mean many things.) We become Chinese medicine practitioners because we wish to be of service. As noble as this may be, it is also a worthy lesson to recognize the contours of what we can do in support of chronic illness patients. Setting boundaries in the interest of both patient and self makes for a healthier, more balanced clinical experience. Being well aware of where Chinese medicine ends and when biomedicine should begin (and vice versa) is a sine qua non. The initial chapter of *Chinese Medicine* outlines parameters related to this very issue and describes the types of patients a clinician may encounter.

We will wish to begin at the beginning. Thus, my focus in chapter two revolves around the subject of our methods of diagnosis and initial intake. For most of us, this encounter does not only focus on the chief complaint. It is also an opportunity to develop our connection with the patient. For some of us, this is quite a long visit. With patients who have mystery diseases and an extraordinarily complex presentation, or diagnosed hypermobile Ehlers-Danlos syndrome (hEDS) and a byzantine array of signs and symptoms, this could mean an extraordinarily long appointment that goes in five directions and gets both parties nowhere. What do we need to know when we conduct an initial intake with someone who has a jaw-dropping list of disorders and dysfunctions? How does a practitioner choose a focus and maintain it but still listen to the patient and leave him or her or them feeling genuinely heard? It may be that the patient has medical post-traumatic stress disorder (PTSD) and the practitioner needs to be aware of not only their story but also how they are embedded within a larger context. There are ways to improve the initial visit for both patient and clinician, and in the second chapter I share clinical pearls to simplify this process.

Working with hEDS means treating an incurable condition that is often progressive and can be debilitating. Understanding the contours of a syndrome that is challenging to treat and harder to live with requires the ability to pick one's battles. In the third chapter, I outline four main ways to begin. Treating the patient for Bi syndrome is one focus. Deciding that the patient is best served by beginning with the Spleen/Stomach as the home base from which all things begin is another option. Addressing physical pain may take second place to a primary focus on treating the shen. If the patient has had Lyme disease or exposure to toxic mold, it might work to reconsider notions of Gu syndrome. A practitioner saves time and energy by choosing a battlefield and working from there. It is too easy to play the medical version of whack-a-mole otherwise. As practitioners, we hope that all roads lead to Beijing (in this case, the patient achieving their best level of optimal health), but a practitioner takes a patient there by choosing wisely and staying on a path. This chapter helps a practitioner to decide which path to take.

Choosing one of the four starting points is but a first step. Working with a complex and systemic disorder requires a nuanced and mindful approach to point selection. In chapter four, I offer insight as to why a practitioner might center zangfu rather than channel or point and vice versa. I also discuss the place of channel theory and the precedence of channel over point. Though there is overlap in each of these themes, the particular needs of an HCTD patient are an invitation to the practitioner to revisit these questions not just once but many times over the course of treatment. I do the same as we move along through each chapter. In addition, I share the more efficacious and safe acupuncture points that a practitioner may select for bodies that are hyperflexible, hyper-reactive, and potentially fragile. How do we remain safe?

Familiarity with this patient population will ultimately make such ponderings less of a requirement and more of a pleasure (for is it not true that Chinese medicine demands excellent critical thinking skills from us all, neophyte and master alike?). My intent with this section is to offer ways to think critically about both the medicine and its delivery in the context of complex cases.

Chapter five is an extension of this theme, and in it, I delineate modalities. As with the preceding chapters, this one reiterates a foundational concept that underpins the entire structure of *Chinese Medicine*. To wit: safe, meaningful, and effective treatment requires knowledge of not the normative body but, instead, the normative body *for a person with hEDS*. Determining what that is when each patient seems to have broken the mold is not easy but it can become intuitive with consistent practice and excellent interpretative skills. It may seem repetitive when I circle back to topics such as diagnosis or pain or each-patient-is-unique as a trope. But by viewing and reviewing these polysemic concepts, we imbibe them fully and are not distracted by difference when it presents in clinic. At times, in response, we use acupuncture needles; otherwise, we try vaccaria seeds. In places, tui na is our best recourse, or perhaps we might opt for cups or another means. In so doing, we respond to the hEDS in all its moveable expressivity, thus demonstrating, once again, the excellence of Chinese medicine and its multiple modalities.

A lifetime of inquiry is made fruitful by guidelines and strategies. But where on earth, when the disorder is so very complicated, do we begin? Where are the touchstones and the guideposts? It can seem irredeemably daunting in the absence of a basic roadmap. In chapter six, consequently, I provide some options for further study. These are not definitive resources but, instead, meant to provide examples of how to go about deepening one's connection with both our medicine and a medical condition that requires considerable agility of thought and broad knowledge at the very minimum. One of the aspects of Chinese medicine that I love is that it is a scholar's medicine if the practitioner chooses that route. But whether or not one wishes to be a scholar-physician, the fact is this: when a practitioner opts to treat complex conditions, they become, by default, scholarly. Cookie-cutter memorization is not enough, even if one has a prodigious memory or is skilled at Google searching.

Over the course of *Chinese Medicine*, we view and review three themes adjacent to the condition itself. The Ehlers-Danlos syndromes are a disorder of connective tissue in the living body. To know them is to also recognize that medicine as it is practiced today suffers its own disorders of connectivity. We cannot understand EDS if we do not investigate the fabric that links us all, the world over, to one another and to our medical traditions. These three recurring themes that provide, after their own fashion, the metaphoric connective tissue for this book relate to concepts surrounding diagnosis, an investigation into ways of seeing, and an analysis of the state of Chinese medicine in professional and global imaginaries. It is here that my background in comparative literature is unmistakable. In essence, "one of our successful strategies is our interdisciplinarity. Comparative literature teaches us to adjust to multiple frames of reference and to attend to relations rather than givens" (Saussy 2006, p.34). In my estimation, none of the aforementioned three themes are comprehensible in the absence of comparison, with one against the other, and by holding *this* alongside *that*.

What may be innovative herein is that I do not hold Western medicine as the normative value against which Chinese therapeutics are compared. For me, Chinese medicine is the home base and the authority against which any *other* is evaluated.

Diagnosis can mean a lot of things. Patients might view this notion as the culmination of a labyrinthine process, one that is a validation; in other instances, it may be a devastating blow. It is a legal concept. Who is granted the authority to diagnose and how do scope-of-practice laws and medical systems make use of the languages of diagnosis? The gap between the research laboratory and the clinical space is enormous. For Western biomedicine, diagnosis aspires to a straight line between symptom and definition, a closure of sorts. For Chinese medicine, diagnosis holds an especially venerated position that, in its elegance, is allusive of the heart of the tradition's very being. I draw from a range of sources in my consideration of this theme. Eric Karchmer's *Prescriptions for Virtuosity: The Postcolonial Struggle of Chinese Medicine* is a touchstone to which I return again and again; equally so are Wang Ju-Yi and Jason Robertson's *Applied Channel Theory in Chinese Medicine: Wang Ju-Yi's Lectures on Channel Therapeutics*, Liu Lihong's *Classical Chinese Medicine*, and Nigel Ching's *The Art and Practice of Diagnosis in Chinese Medicine*. Western biomedicine is not immune to debate regarding diagnosis and thus I make use of sources from within its traditions as well.

Clause 1-1 of *Synopsis of Prescriptions of the Golden Chamber* begins with a question, "Would you kindly explain the meaning of 'A superior doctor will cure a disease before its onset'?" (Zhang 1987, p.2). There are many legendary anecdotes about prowess that entail seeing below the surface. These narratives serve to bolster our rightful pride in Chinese medicine as the ultimate form of preventative healthcare. They also demonstrate a value system that privileges a scholarly, almost superhuman capacity to discern, predict, and redirect the course of disease. I return to these stories within the tissues of this book and present them with the invitation to revisit our ideas of seeing. Chinese medicine is a medicine of deeply seeing and delivering nuanced strategies to unearth root cause and change the course of its effects.

But chapter two of *Su Wen* concludes with a question that resonates:

> Now,
> when drugs are employed for therapy only after a disease has
> become fully
> developed,
> when [attempts at] restoring order are initiated only after the
> disorder has fully developed,
> this is as if a well were dug when one is thirsty,
> and as if weapons were cast when the fight is on.
> Would this not be too late, too? (Unschuld 1986, p.57)

In many ways, it is too late. The first quarter of the twenty-first century winds to its conclusion in a world marked by a global pandemic. Rates of autoimmune disease are increasing apace. EDS and other debilitating syndromes are proliferating. As I argue throughout *Chinese Medicine*, there are ways to see that respond directly to our current challenges. We take recourse in our classical ancestors to be sure. But what that means to our patients within our clinics and to our identities as practitioners has shifted in response to the challenges we now face. A recurring theme herein, consequently, is an invitation to question how it is that we see.

Chinese medicine is now a world medicine. This is, at heart, the root cause of some of our discontent and it is equally a metaphoric center. The imaginary of China and what constitutes authentic Chinese medicine is akin to the very *ming men* that provides us with ministerial fire to energize our journeys. The venerable home country of this beloved medicine underwent its own conflicts as it decided whether and how to maintain indigenous tradition as a pillar of its healthcare and cultural identities. To trace Chinese medicine's history is beyond the scope of this book. But we cannot ignore it, either. How patients see us, why they come to us for support, how laws and systems and shifts in perception affect us, the practitioners, and our patients...who are we and how, in fact, do we learn? What, if we ponder it, is Chinese medicine? Where, if we are far from Beijing, do we find our center? All of these questions thread through *Chinese Medicine*. Their answers make a difference to the ways in which we engage with mystery-disease patients and complex disorders like EDS.

One thing I know for sure: we look for relations, not givens, and in this way, we develop a fluid and fluent language of HCTDs as treated by Chinese medicine. We look and we look again, and what we see broadens our horizons exponentially. We see ourselves perhaps the way we might view Spanish along the southern borders of the United States: as a borderlands territory, one that thrives and grows and has long since developed ways of communicating, one that takes from more than one language or tradition. The practitioner benefits and so does the patient when we interrogate our notions of subjectivity as practitioners of Chinese medicine who may or may not be from China. My call to arms in the final section is that each of us in the profession stretches a bit. Whether the reader of this project is monocultural or multicultural, whether fluent in Chinese or not, we can all benefit when we expand our horizons. We can all benefit from a view and re-view of what the practice of Chinese medicine looks like when it is applied in a clinical setting for the benefit of patients with so-called rare diseases.

Asking the proverbial fish what water is like will not elicit useful information; even if the fish spoke English (or Spanish or Chinese or Italian or…), it still remains too close to its roots to know what is and is not remarkable about the substance that provides its oxygen. The amount of information that is poured upon a student of Chinese medicine is prodigious. Clinical experience after becoming licensed adds to that bank of knowledge. Continuing education requirements may be a useful supplement to knowledge, but that can depend on what is available. It is my professional opinion that there are gaps in how we are taught to approach this medicine.

The world is a bigger place when we hop out of our proverbial fishbowls and experience the texture of waters not our own.

Being able to place ourselves within our individual subject positions and having the self-awareness to interrogate our received wisdom is a worthy task. The goal of the final chapter of *Chinese Medicine* is to provide guidelines. What each reader does with this material will be individual to that person. My hope is that it will prove useful not just for treating HCTD but also for deepening one's connection with Chinese medicine.

It is daunting to treat patients with hEDS. Not even Hua Tuo himself, nor Sun Si Miao, or even Li Gao could have cured this condition. But we can ameliorate the suffering it causes. Chinese medicine is a profound healing medicine. We take the slightest glimmer of wellbeing potential and nurture its flame so that whatever is there, we make it glow. We rely on a treasure house of precedence when we strengthen digestion or calm shen or lessen pain. If we are excellent communicators on an intercultural level, we can help patients in need to engage more fruitfully with their biomedical care providers. An hEDS patient may only come to us for a limited part of their healthcare or we may be their primary resource. Either way, we make a difference. We do so by standing on the shoulders of giants.

Let us begin, now, this journey of a thousand steps.

# CHAPTER 1

# A Hydra

## I. What Are the Ehlers-Danlos Syndromes? (A Detailed Sketch)

The Hydra, as we will recollect, is the nine-headed daughter of Typhon and Echidna of Greek mythology, and Hercules is tasked with slaying her as the second of his twelve labors. This is no easy feat, given that when he cuts off one head two more appear in response. Until he removes the dominant one, there is no possibility of success. Getting to the root of the problem seems all but impossible and this task is but the start of a series of twelve challenges set before him. With assistance and bolstered by destiny, Hercules does complete this second labor and is able to advance to the third task and the subsequent nine remaining. Determination, fate, and a certain level of luck form his path; ultimately, Hercules succeeds in his quest and anyone in confrontation with metaphorical versions of such challenges might do the same. The short answer to the question above is that EDS, or Ehlers-Danlos syndrome, is a genetically determined connective tissue disorder. The longer, more realistic narrative is that this is, as it is correctly termed, the Ehlers-Danlos syndromes, plural, and that it is a medical hydra of prodigious contour.

But what does this mean? How is parsing the vagaries of a complicated genetic dysfunction relevant to the practice of Chinese medicine? Why begin with the biomedical narrative?

Beyond the obvious (patient safety and our need to remain within our scope of practice), there are specific reasons why we might begin this way. As I demonstrate over the course of this book, we can expect quite a lot from Chinese medicine when it comes to the treatment of our Ehlers-Danlos patients. When we understand what biomedicine does and is capable of doing for people with EDS, we can appreciate allopathic systems and then determine what Chinese medicine can contribute. When we recognize where biomedicine falls short, we look to our profession with self-awareness and note where we might take up the task of serving patients. There are some areas where scientific findings are fairly clear-cut and there are others that are murky. When we know the terrain, we are able to determine where our unique strengths lie within it. As I argue, disorders of connective tissue will become more common in upcoming decades. The more we know, the more effectively and safely we are able to treat patients.

Hypermobile Ehlers-Danlos syndrome, or hEDS, is not rare, not really, and it will become recognized as being less aberrant as time passes.[1] Awareness of comorbid conditions associated with EDS, including mast cell activation syndrome (MCAS), is slowly disseminating through the public imaginary and within medical establishments. By understanding current narratives, we become multilingual in terms of connective tissue disorder. We do not need to become amateur histologists to understand EDS but it is worthwhile to review the foundations of this condition. Whether or not it is new (or long-forgotten) information for us, we focus on the ground level when we begin at the beginning. The tissues and their genetic makeup are where it all starts. This is also useful material to keep in mind when educating patients about the scientific basis of their lived experience. Patients want to understand what is happening with their bodies and, although people with hEDS are often extremely good at recognizing and defining their ailments, it is still helpful to be able to reduce all themes involved to their simplest parameters.

A brief overview starts at the micro-level. We of course remember that collections of interconnected cells are called biological tissues and that the human body is made up of four primary types, namely: epithelial (surface and glandular), muscle (contractile cells), nervous (neurons and glial cells), and connective, which provides material for both form and function throughout the entire body. Connective tissue cells are loosely packed in an extracellular matrix that consists of ground substances and fibers, the most important of which is collagen. This is a hardworking substance. Not only does this tissue support its corporeal colleagues. In addition, cells associated with immune defense are housed within connective tissue. As a component of nearly every organ, its tasks are multiple. The ubiquity of connective tissue is a testament to labyrinthine possibilities when assessing an Ehlers-Danlos patient's presentation.

And what of this extracellular matrix? One of its primary components, the aforementioned collagen, is the most abundant protein in the body and there are different varieties of it in varying areas from top to toe. Type I collagen is a component of the skin, tendons, ligaments, and fascia. Tendons and ligaments are made primarily of Type I collagen, with elastin making up a smaller percentage of their content. Type VI pertains to the smooth and skeletal muscle fibers, and dysfunction related to this form expresses via muscle weakness and dystrophy. Collagen, a relatively yin substance, provides tensile strength to the structure in question. A related fiber, elastin, is another protein substance found within the extracellular matrix and its function is (as its name suggests) to provide flexibility. Relatively yang, elastin pertains to the element of stretching out and returning to a quiescent starting state. Together, collagen and elastin are essential to skin, large arteries, lungs, tendons, and cartilage.

To have a genetic alteration that throws a wrench into the process of making or using collagen means different things to different bodies and requires different therapeutic approaches in response. Connective tissue is a foundation of the body, and EDS as a result can affect just about any aspect or system associated with it. As much as I have tried to be brief in this chapter, there is a lot to cover. In the final chapter of *Chinese Medicine*, consequently, I took great care to provide valuable resources for further investigation.

A practitioner who is known for treating hEDS patients will soon build a roster of patients with connective tissue dysfunction, and it is necessary to be able to differentiate between them. It is useful to remember the differences between the acronyms CTD, HCTD, and MCTD. CTD, or connective tissue *disease*, can be understood to refer to autoimmune disease, with some of the more common ones being rheumatoid arthritis, scleroderma, systemic lupus erythematosus (SLE), polymyositis, and dermatomyositis. CTD differs from *heritable* connective tissue *disorder* (HCTD), which includes a range of conditions and levels of disability. These would be the Ehlers-Danlos syndromes, Marfan syndrome, osteogenesis imperfecta, and other rare conditions such as Loeys-Dietz syndrome. Mixed connective tissue disease, or MCTD, is also known as Sharp's syndrome and it is a distinct rheumatic condition that entails multiple CTDs. These can include the aforementioned lupus, scleroderma, polymyositis, and even EDS on top of all of it. Yes, a person with a genetic dysfunction of the connective tissue, or HCTD, can also develop autoimmune disease, or CTD.

My description of these categories gives an appearance of simplicity that is deceptive. There is little about these conditions that can be considered uncomplicated, and, for many, the obstacle course begins when a patient sets out to find a diagnosis. And yet, there are degrees of challenge in comparing one alongside the other. The CTD patient with an autoimmune condition will generally fit within a relatively stable diagnostic category (the key word being "relatively"). People with HCTDs will often have comorbid conditions and fluctuating signs and symptoms that make diagnosis considerably more challenging. MCTD, for its part, can be just as puzzling and complex as the Ehlers-Danlos syndromes. Once diagnosed (or if diagnosed), there is often a proliferation of other difficulties, for none of these conditions are easy to treat. In some instances, biomedical intervention is unequivocally the safer and more effective approach; in others, Chinese medicine is certainly better. At times, either/or could be equally valid and, of course, a combined approach can be optimal in many instances. A lot depends on the patient, their access to healthcare, and the degree to which their individual presentation affects their life.

Hypermobile EDS, or hEDS, is one of fourteen subtypes within the larger umbrella of the Ehlers-Danlos syndromes, and it is the only one without an officially identified genetic marker at present. Histology's story is parsed via laboratory research undertaken by geneticists. Research findings and genetic testing in contemporary biomedicine have rewritten much of the narratives surrounding HCTDs as they are viewed today, and the lack of a known genetic determinant for hEDS causes ripples in a multitude of spheres.[2] However, as I demonstrate over the course of *Chinese Medicine*, current knowledge is continuously expanding and what we accept as received wisdom today might be displaced tomorrow by new findings. But patients will remain patients, and the core need to reduce pain and anxiety and to ameliorate the challenges wrought by these conditions will stay the same. How well we can address these core needs depends on the ability to think critically and to apply our knowledge mindfully.

It is helpful to recollect the differences between inheritance patterns. Some of the variations are autosomal dominant, so even if only one parent has a copy of the defective gene, the offspring can still inherit it. Others are autosomal recessive, so both parents must carry the gene and the chances of their child being born with the condition are one in four. When we consider what sort of genetic misfiring occurs with these defects, the possibilities include dysfunction stemming from collagen structure or processing in the body and/or there can be missteps in the folding and cross-linking of intracellular processes related to the collagen.[3] And while the Ehlers-Danlos syndromes across the board are characterized by joint hypermobility, skin hyperextensibility, and tissue fragility, each individual version has its own genetic defect and resulting presentation that then determines where it is placed within one of what are currently fourteen identified subtypes.[4]

While considering the biomedical narrative of this disease, it is worthwhile to note that classification of the Ehlers-Danlos syndromes as a disease (in other words, nosology) currently looks at the genetic markers associated with it (the genotypes) and the symptoms as they appear in the embodied experience of the patient (in other words, the phenotype). Classification has shifted over the course of the past thirty or so years and is, at the time of this writing, not entirely stable. New research is even now expanding the parameters of these categories, and what is most useful, I think, is to consider how the narratives have been constructed over the course of time. I address this issue briefly here and return to it at the end of this chapter. Because it is such an important key to the understanding of the lived experience of EDS, I will return to it in the final chapter of *Chinese Medicine*.

How illnesses, especially complex ones without clear boundaries or fixed protocols surrounding their treatment, are discovered, named, and categorized has a trickle-down effect that shapes patients and how they navigate within the confines of their conditions. Looking at the how-did-we-get-here question requires a review of the history and an interrogation of the present and future.

The recognition that some people are more flexible than others has been noted since the time of Hippocrates, but it was not until 1901 and 1908 that Edvard Ehlers and Henri-Alexandre Danlos, respectively, established their definitive outlines of the condition that bears their names. In 1936, this collagen disorder was designated as the Ehlers-Danlos syndromes. The 1960s were a time of considerable research and discovery, while the period between 1988 and 2017 saw three substantive modifications of classification, each more refined than its predecessor. Science's goal in this context is to link genotype and phenotype in order to identify subtypes and to provide better treatments to patients. In 1988, the Berlin nosology expanded the number of subtypes of EDS from five to eleven. The Villefranche adaption of 1997 reduced this number to six subtypes. Current guidelines published by the International Consortium on the Ehlers-Danlos Syndromes in 2017 revised the Villefranche nosology and expanded the number of subtypes to thirteen.

Of the subtypes, only hEDS remains marginalized by definitions granted by genetic identification, though advances in research will more likely than not soon change this status. Currently, though, its diagnosis relies on clinical presentation and a set list of criteria. The 2017 shift in diagnostic markers for people with hEDS has caused bitterness in the hypermobile community and has been viewed by some as an act of moving goalposts that excludes people from being diagnosed.

To complicate the issue, medicine also acknowledges hypermobility along a spectrum. Though not necessarily benign, the nomenclature for a remarkably flexible person without joint pain used to be called "benign joint hypermobility syndrome" (BJHS). Current iterations categorize such presentations as hypermobility spectrum disorders (HSD), and some consider it to be essentially the same thing as hEDS. My experience with patients who have what would be considered HSD is that it is not always a benign condition. Especially if a patient is hypermobile-plus (in other words, hypermobile plus they have comorbid conditions), the distinction between hEDS and BJHS or HSD is academic. The lived experience of the patient from one to the other might not be different at all.

However, gene mutations associated with hEDS have been identified and research findings continuously shift narratives. In addition, there are some fascinating ideas regarding the immune system's role in collagen dysfunction, not to mention others pertaining to metabolism of folate. I address these and other theories over the course of this book. Before veering onto the subject of current scientific developments, it is helpful to outline a larger picture. We will probably not ever see most of the subtypes I am about to present but, if we wish to treat HCTDs, then we need to know of them. It is not possible to understand hEDS without an understanding of the subtypes. Furthermore, we cannot adequately treat patients with HCTDs if we do not know about comorbidities associated with EDS. The following section is a bit of a laundry list and it may also seem daunting. But it is a summary of what we all need to know and is not intended to discourage anyone.

When one begins, it is surprising how many variations one actually sees in clinic. As time goes by and experience becomes deepened and more mature, it becomes second nature to knowledgeably navigate the vagaries of connective tissue. Bodies are complex miracles, even when they are problematic and cause suffering to their inhabitants.

## II. One More Time... What Are the Ehlers-Danlos Syndromes?

Detailing all the different variants of EDS is counterproductive. Instead, it helps us to better understand the syndrome if we are familiar with the basic concepts I share via a brief sketch. We also need to be aware of the comorbid conditions associated with EDS and I outline them in this chapter and discuss them in the context of Chinese medicine throughout this book.

We do not need to memorize subtypes. In fact, many primary

care providers (PCPs) either do not know much about the full range of subtypes and their attendant comorbidities or they are not confident about their degree of familiarity with the syndrome as a whole.[5] However, when we possess a general awareness of the currently identified subtypes, we are fulfilling our baseline professional obligation if we expect to meaningfully treat HCTD patients. We might follow up and investigate further, and I offer suggestions for that in the final chapter of *Chinese Medicine*. But unless we intend to return to medical school to become geneticists or rheumatologists, we can opt for an overview, rather than a detailed account of the types of EDS that are currently identified. Consequently, the outlines I provide include only salient information.[6]

These are the thirteen subtypes included in the International Consortium on the Ehlers-Danlos Syndromes 2017 list:

- Classical EDS (cEDS) focuses on the skin and requires a specific level of dermal hyperextensibility plus atrophic scarring and generalized joint hypermobility (GJH) for diagnosis.

- Classical-like EDS (clEDS) presentations involve hyperextensible skin with velvety texture and absence of atrophic scars, GJH that may include repeated dislocations (usually shoulder or ankle), and easily bruised skin or unexplained discoloration due to subsurface bleeding (spontaneous ecchymoses).

- Cardiac-valvular EDS (cvEDS) is a rare type that presents with skin issues similar to the above-noted, plus joint hypermobility that can manifest throughout the body or be confined to the small joints. The main concern of this subtype is that it includes severe and progressive cardiac and valvular problems that affect the aortic and mitral valves.

- Vascular EDS (vEDS) is diagnosed based on family history

and events such as arterial rupture at a young age in addition to spontaneous ruptures in other systems, such as the sigmoid colon or the uterus during pregnancy in the third trimester, and carotid-cavernous sinus fistula (CCSF) formation without a preceding trauma.

- Hypermobile EDS (hEDS) is thought to be the most common type and constitutes the focus of this book. Criteria for diagnosis will be addressed in greater detail subsequent to this list.

- Arthrochalasia EDS (aEDS) is determined based on factors including congenital hip dislocation, a history of severe GJH with repeated or many subluxations, and skin hyperextensibility.

- Dermatosparaxis EDS (dEDS) identification rests upon nine major criteria and eleven minor signs, including the presence of extreme skin fragility and notable craniofacial features.

- Kyphoscoliotic EDS (kEDS) is a form that is seen with congenital muscle hypotonia, progressive or non-progressive scoliosis that is present at birth or which shows an early onset, and a pattern of GJH that is mainly in the shoulders, hips, and knees.

- Brittle cornea syndrome (BCS) is descriptive. The patient has thin corneas and experiences early onset and progressive keratoconus (thinning, bulging corneas that progress as the patient ages) or keratoglobus (the same, only present at birth) plus blue sclerae.

- Spondylodysplastic EDS (spEDS) is another rare subtype that is characterized by short stature, muscle hypotonia, and bowed legs.

- Musculocontractural EDS (mcEDS) is determined by criteria that include multiple congenital contractures (adduction-flexion and/or clubfoot), specific craniofacial features present at birth or evident in early infancy, and skin features such as hyperflexibility, easy bruising, fragility with atrophic scars, and increased palmar wrinkling.

- Myopathic EDS (mEDS) is a subtype that involves congenital muscle hypotonia and/or atrophy that improves with age, a history of proximal joint contractures (notably the knee, hip, and/or elbow), and hypermobility of the distal joints.

- Periodontal EDS (pEDS) manifests in the gums with intractable gingivitis, lack of attachment in the gingiva, and brownish-yellow shin lesions (pretibial plaques).

At this point, a reader might be wondering how this information supports a Chinese medicine practitioner's understanding of this disorder. Do we need to be tethered by the narratives of evidenced-based medicine and the tyranny of the gene? As with anything related to Chinese medicine, the answer to all questions is both yes and no. For some of us, evidence-based conclusions are the sine qua non. For others, less so or maybe even not at all. Chinese medicine does not require knowledge of genetics. However, it does behoove us to be aware of up-to-date findings and past narratives. In so doing, a practitioner can help their patients to navigate a siloed Western biomedical system. An astute clinician might observe red-flag symptoms that need follow-up with the allopathic practitioner. In the case of EDS, whichever subtype it might be, a knowledge of how biomedicine finds it, narrates it, and treats it is the equivalent of being bilingual and multicultural once refracted through the lens and languages of Chinese medicine.

Most practitioners, whether or not they are aware of it, have treated an hEDS patient, and some of us realize that we are amongst the ranks of the hypermobile in so doing. When I undertook yoga teacher training in 2012, for example, I started to become aware of the distinction between not flexible, relatively normal flexibility, and potentially dangerous joint laxity degrees of flexible. Though I had considerable experience with gym culture and practice, I looked back and realized that my own hyperflexibility was so normal to me that I did not pay attention to it in others. Becoming certified to teach Hatha yoga changed that, even though I did not launch a career as a yoga teacher. Instead, that year, I started my program in Chinese medicine and soon discovered tui na, which taught me more than I had ever dreamed about the tangible expression of a wide variety of hypermobile bodies. Later, in student clinic, I attracted patients who suffered from joint problems, hyperflexibility, and pain. At that point, I started to look at my own history with a genuinely altered perspective.

By now, having built my practice in large measure on the treatment of CTDs and HCTDs, I have a different knowledge of these conditions and how my patients (and indeed I myself) fit within them. The same will be true of anyone who builds a practice that supports connective tissue wellbeing.

Again: most practitioners will have treated patients with hEDS and, beyond that, many of us have seen cases of Marfan syndrome and MCTD, whether or not we recognized it at the time. Most of us, especially if this book is as useful as I hope it to be, will treat these conditions and become familiar with the vagaries of connective tissue dysfunction as HCTDs become more and more prominent in both the cultural imaginary and the clinical space. Yes, it is a hydra, and yes, when dealing with hydras, it is useful to have recourse to multiple systems of understanding. How these narratives are constructed and why they are set up the way that they are may seem byzantine or even boring, especially if one has little or no connection with biomedicine.

It is not boring though. It is not. Instead, the genetic narrative surrounding each subtype is a living history that delineates many of the contours of what our patients experience. They live within their bodies but their bodies live within these systems, as do we all.

The Berlin and Villefranche nosologies that are now replaced by the 2017 International Consortium on the Ehlers-Danlos Syndromes are not the only accounts outlining EDS and other HCTDs. It is instructive to look at a landmark written by Victor A. McKusick, an American researcher sometimes referred to as the father of American medical genetics. *Heritable Disorders of Connective Tissue*, originally published in 1960, has been reprinted multiple times and continues to be relevant. Online booksellers being what they are, I managed to acquire a copy of one of the oldest versions of this volume, the third reprint of 1966. Comparing it with recent iterations of the text was painful. The way disabled bodies are presented in 1960s-era medical books is sobering. The photographs show individuals who are set in front of measuring marks like criminals in an old-fashioned police line-up. The stories describing them in case study format tell of great depths of suffering. What is tangible and visible, the phenotype, is painstakingly collected in these earliest accounts, and what is demonstrated therein is striking and deeply poignant.

It truly is worth comparing the current nosology against earlier versions if one is so inclined to discover just how wide-ranging this condition can be and what, given scientific knowledge, is included or discarded. As I discuss later in this chapter and in the final section of *Chinese Medicine*, there are emerging theories regarding hEDS that will probably result in a new nosology and number of subtypes.

But I get ahead of myself.

Broadly speaking, a practitioner of Chinese medicine is more likely to have patients with hEDS or undiagnosed variants of the Ehlers-Danlos syndromes or other genetic conditions such as Marfan syndrome than patients with the other versions of EDS. It is useful to know what the biomedical community is finding, reporting, and doing if only due to the ubiquity of hypermobility as a broad category. Leading researchers and patients alike lament the lack of knowledge of connective tissue disorders. However, the more experience we have with hypermobile patients, the more we begin to notice that more and more routine pain patients show signs of connective tissue disorder. Other cases, such as digestive complaints that previously were seen as food sensitivity or allergy, are something else, maybe MCAS. There is a tremendous range of what might be considered normal and within a reference range deemed healthy, but the same can be said for the opposite.

Some of the Western biomedical narrative is easily translatable to Chinese medicine's terms and other aspects of it are not. The translatable aspects I reserve for subsequent chapters of this book. I consider the parts that do not exchange well with our profession in this chapter for two reasons. First, this is a disorder that does have a complete language via biomedicine and patients navigate within it as their primary territory (for the most part). Common sense makes it clear where to begin, and that is with the biomedical narrative. This becomes especially significant when we consider issues related to patient safety. We need to know how to identify red flags. Second, it is important to consider how multilingualism in healthcare expands one's horizons. Reading a text in my own native language is one way of imbibing literature. If I read in another language, one not my own, the reading is enriched by taking that narrative on its own terms, by comparing it with my native language, and by going back once again to the work in its original. The act of engaging in comparison and contrast deepens one's knowledge when one reads literature. The same can be said for studying biomedicine alongside one's Chinese medical texts as we develop skill in reading narratives of the patient's condition as it presents in clinic.

Though we may tend to begin from the starting point of hypermobile joints or remarkable laxity of skin, such signs or symptoms are in no way the endpoint. Any form of EDS has multiple manifestations and can present inconsistently. Symptoms that come and go from one day to the next or even which change by the hour and which are not amenable to diagnosis make it challenging to determine cause and effect. What we know, via the above-sketched outline, compared with what we might see in clinic make my digressions herein clear: this is a hydra. We begin with an outline and we learn, in clinic, about variations and the lived experiences of our patients. It is a process that requires time, experience, patience, and curiosity.

We might begin by asking ourselves if we remember learning about this condition in our Western medicine coursework. If an allopathic physician has heard of this condition, their familiarity with it might not extend past a vague memory of the tried-and-true photograph of a contortionist in their medical school textbook. This is not a lacuna in Western biomedical knowledge unshared by Chinese medicine practitioners. We did not focus on this clichéd textbook depiction in the biomedical track of my program. I do remember feeling very sorry for the figure in the picture and wondering how badly his joints hurt after he untangled them from around his neck. I remember that I thought his eyes looked sad. But we did not dedicate any class discussion to that picture during my anatomy and physiology classes. Yet I was haunted by that picture, though I knew not why at the time, and when I began to treat patients in student clinic, I remembered the figure of the contortionist and went back to it. He had EDS, the description beneath him said, and that was all I needed to begin a course of study that will probably occupy a good part of the rest of my life.

A picture is worth a thousand words, no doubt, and it is a reminder to continue to press, to continue to study, and to continue to learn. A patient can be injured by a physical therapist

(PT) who does not know enough about connective tissue disorder. A chiropractor can inflict serious damage on this population. So, unfortunately, can a Chinese medicine practitioner. Western biomedicine and scientific research do not have all the answers to the hydra that is the Ehlers-Danlos syndromes. Nor does any other medical tradition. The more multilingual a practitioner is, the better we can determine what our practice can do and what, outside of that, is due for a referral. This condition stretches well beyond the parameters of joints and ligaments. A significant aspect of its burdens comes from a patient's medical mysteries and consequent struggle to find appropriate and meaningful healthcare. As the following section makes clear, there is much more to this condition than simply joint laxity, soft skin, and recalcitrant collagen.

## III. But That's Not All: MCAS, POTS, Chiari, Tethered Cord, Dysautonomia, Prolapse, Anxiety, Autism, Marfan Syndrome... (A Summary of Adjacent Issues)

Working with hEDS rarely confines itself to just the matter of connective tissue and the joints. It is likely that a patient lives with at least one if not many more of the following common comorbidities that I outline here. The two most common comorbidities are postural orthopedic tachycardia syndrome, or POTS, and mast cell activation syndrome, or MCAS. When medical care providers and people in the EDS community speak of "the trifecta," they are referencing hEDS, POTS, and MCAS.[7] When we routinely treat hEDS patients we become very familiar with POTS and MCAS. Other conditions might be less common in our clinics but we still need to know of them for the sake of patient safety. Chinese medicine can at the very least ameliorate many of these disorders, to be sure, and approaches and modalities are the subject of subsequent chapters. Within the context of a discussion of biomedicine in this chapter, though, it is useful to acquire some basic information and practical knowledge.

So it begins...

It is unsurprising that **POTS** is a common comorbidity for hEDS patients.[8] What is puzzling, instead, is how challenging it can be to get diagnosed. A hallmark of this condition is a heart rate increase of 30 beats per minute (BPM) in adults and 40 BPM in adolescents when going from sitting to standing, and symptoms can include sweatiness, shaking, brain fog, exhaustion, fainting, or dizziness when changing position. This is due to blood pooling in the extremities and the body's inability to adequately move said fluid towards the brain and upper body upon changing posture. Though patients may have a hard time getting an official diagnosis, people do tend to know when they have it and my experience is that a new patient will at least know to tell me that they faint easily. This is important to keep in mind in order to avoid instances of needle shock; as with patients who have dysautonomia, it is wise to start with a light hand until we know how they react to acupuncture treatment.

Timing is also a consideration. I ask at the initial appointment how much time a patient may need in order to transition from treatment table to standing and being ready to depart. In response, patients have shared anecdotes about being at other medical offices and getting berated for not being able to get up and go when the appointment should have concluded. There is a real sense of shame and anger at this treatment. A person with POTS can't help it when they are unable to stand and exit the treatment room. I had a patient, once, who had to lie down on the floor for almost ten minutes before slowly moving to sitting and then slowly, slowly moving to standing. Fortunately, I had the space to allow them an extra twenty minutes, but I learned from that and other similar experiences to ask about transition time.

Mast cells are immune cells found throughout connective tissue, and dysregulation of these cells is relatively common in HCTD populations. **MCAS** occurs when the immune system cells degranulate improperly, either too often or too vigorously. The root cause of this condition is unknown but patients with it experience repeated episodes of anaphylaxis in response to even the mildest of stimuli. When mast cells detect a trigger, be it medication, an insect bite, food, an odor, or other, they release histamine and other mast cell mediators into the blood stream, thus wreaking havoc of protean contour. MCAS is becoming more and more commonly seen in our clinics and there are many more factors involved than just that which is wrought by connective tissue disorder.[9]

**Histamine intolerance** is a subset of MCAS. A Chinese medicine practitioner is likely to see patients who present with mold toxicity issues that result in histamine intolerance. One might also see patients with Lyme disease and its long-term consequences that include histamine intolerance. This is not MCAS's gentler cousin. It can be difficult to manage. However, MCAS is much more variable and wide-ranging. A true case of MCAS can be associated with everything from asthma, candida overgrowth, chronic inflammatory response syndrome (CIRS), infertility, endometriosis, and more. When we have a patient with EDS who is inflamed by everything and reactive to pretty much anything, this is probably MCAS rather than histamine intolerance.[10]

We need to be aware of the signs and symptoms of MCAS when we work with HCTDs. Not every patient requires biomedical intervention for MCAS, but many do. This will depend on the individual. The very least a Chinese medicine practitioner who works with EDS must do is maintain awareness of signs, symptoms, and red flags. This is a protean condition that can mimic many other diseases and cause or exacerbate a plethora of illnesses. We are best served by maintaining a no-perfume policy (I think that most of us already do) and, if we offer moxibustion, we might consider whether or not we wish to treat patients with HCTDs. A person who suffers from overactive mast cells might experience an alarming reaction to the smell of burning herbs.

**Dysautonomia** is common in EDS patients. This is a dysfunction of the autonomic nervous system that can affect the entire system or just parts of it. Signs and symptoms can include an abnormally fast or slow heart rate, difference in the size of the pupils, difficulty urinating, inability to regulate body temperature, anxiety, headaches, insomnia, constant thirst, and much more. In some patients, POTS may be the only form of dysautonomia that causes undue challenge. In others, it may be much more widespread and debilitating. We are able support a patient and help them to live a better life with dysautonomia, though our role in treating such patients may be limited, depending on severity. Although this depends on the presentation, it is either the neurologist or cardiologist who will diagnose and manage dysautonomia in an EDS patient.

**Gastroparesis**, or incomplete stomach emptying, can be caused by dysautonomia, certain medicines, and/or chronic stress. This can present as GERD or acid reflux, bloating, nausea, feeling full after eating very little, loss of appetite, unexpected weight loss, and difficulty controlling blood sugar. Other gastrointestinal (GI) issues that a practitioner will treat with EDS patients are **irritable bowel syndrome (IBS)**, **constipation**, and various **allergies and sensitivities** that may be part of a larger MCAS picture. Helping a patient to be able to enjoy food and digest it reasonably well is one area where we in Chinese medicine can truly be of service. **Celiac disease** and **gluten intolerance** are common in EDS patients. Parsing whether or not this food allergy is actually a matter of gastroparesis, whether it is a sensitivity, or if it is related to dysautonomia is more of a challenge. However, Chinese medicine for any of these digestive concerns can provide genuinely excellent results.

Functional issues that get in the way of enjoyable eating can also be problematic. **Temporomandibular joint disorder**, or **TMJ disorder**, is fairly common with EDS. Either the joint slips out of place or it locks.

**Drug sensitivity** or a polar opposite can be a factor for EDS patients and when we prescribe herbs or any supplement, we need to be aware of this detail. Herbal safety is a particularly important issue for patients with vEDS, who must take special care with blood thinners and other anticoagulant drugs. How a patient metabolizes different medications can be unique to each individual and so is the way that they absorb topicals. A practitioner who ignores a patient's concerns about dosage does so at their own peril. At best, the patient will lose trust in the practitioner and at worst, the patient will have an extreme or shocking reaction to the herbs. There is a mantra in the EDS community, "low and slow," and it exists for a reason. If we want to be safe, we start with the lowest possible dosage and we move slowly.

**Ptosis and prolapse** are a spectrum. Ptosis is when a structure droops and it is commonly known in reference to eyes although, with EDS patients, this can also occur internally with organs. EDS patients may present with visible ptosis in the eye region. We might also see it in the very droopy skin of a cEDS case. Prolapse, for its part, is the unpleasant experience of having a body part (rectum, bladder, uterus, or vagina) fall out of place. This happens to people whether or not they have connective tissue disorder but it is notably common in people with EDS. My experience with EDS patients who have prolapsed organs is that they resolve this via surgery or under the direction of their urogynecologist. Beforehand, we can help our patients to stave off surgery (if that is what they want), and after, if surgery is unavoidable, we can support them as they recover.

**Median arcuate ligament syndrome** (**MALS**) is when the arc-shaped band of tissue on the chest is tight or otherwise able to press against the celiac artery where it then disrupts blood flow to the internal organs. Patients with MALS will feel pain after eating and develop food aversion. They also experience nausea, bloating, and diarrhea. Usually, this is diagnosed by their medical doctor (MD). When an EDS patient presents with these symptoms, we might ask them if the pain goes away when they lean forward and, if the patient responds in the affirmative, we send them to their doctor straightaway.

**Nutcracker syndrome** is a compression disorder of the aorta and superior mesenteric artery. It is not uncommon for hEDS patients, and PCPs do not always know much about it. People in online EDS communities support each other with information when their doctors do not. I am careful about weighing in with a medical opinion in such venues, but one post touched me and I did comment. The questioner described flank pain, urinary discomfort, and blood in their urine that their PCP had tested and screened and not been able to resolve. They were distressed and feeling gaslit. By the time I wrote, "Have you asked your doctor about nutcracker syndrome?" someone else had chimed in with, "This sounds exactly like me, and I have nutcracker syndrome." A similar condition is floating kidney, and what is happening is just what it sounds like. The kidney drops and compresses the left renal vein, not only leading to flank pain and hematuria—it can also present with pelvic congestion, pain during sexual intercourse in women, and varicose veins in the lower abdomen.

MALS and nutcracker syndrome both require surgery and can be life-threatening if not treated in a timely fashion. A practitioner who has an EDS patient with any of these symptoms can do them a service by educating them so that they can go to their MD with useful information.

**Fibromuscular dysplasia (FMD)** is a condition where the arteries either become stiff or overly loose (stenosis vs. aneurism). Some people can live their whole lives with this condition and not know it; others will experience alarming vascular events as a result of it.[11]

**Pelvic health** concerns include **endometriosis, difficult pregnancy** and **spontaneous abortion**, and **dyspareunia**. EDS can also affect men's pelvic floor health, and **erectile dysfunction** can be problematic. EDS and Marfan syndrome patients show a 30% greater incidence of low testosterone.[12] I have found that relatively younger guys who come in for ED treatment can have a number of signs and symptoms of hEDS if not Marfan syndrome. The 30% greater incidence that I mention is not an abstraction for me; rather, my clinical experience has demonstrated this to be relevant.

**Chiari malformations** involve structural disorders of the base of the skull and the cerebellum. These are graded from I to V, with I being the least severe and V the most. In its most benign presentation, the cerebellum might protrude or be pulled slightly down into the foramen magnum. In its most extreme, there is an incomplete cerebellum and part of the spine or skull might be visible. Chiari is associated with hEDS. In its less-severe manifestations, Chiari may cause dizziness, tinnitus, neck pain, nausea, breathing problems, insomnia, depression, scoliosis, balance issues, and/or muscle weakness and pain. Chiari I is often diagnosed in adulthood, and in all its gradients is treated via surgery. Though usually a congenital condition, it can be triggered by injury or infection. Untreated, Chiari can cause build-up of cerebrospinal fluid that could lead to brain damage.

My experience is that the patients I have treated with Chiari already knew about it when they came to me. However, when we have a patient with an unstable neck who complains of pain after sneezing or coughing, or who has a number of issues (for example scoliosis and tinnitus and a troubled neck), it is a good idea to ask if their medical team has spoken to them about Chiari. An unstable neck requires extra care and knowledge. Sometimes, our tinnitus patient really has something else, something that needs screening and maybe surgery.

**Tethered cord** is a functional and neurological disorder. The caudal aspect of the spinal cord is attached to the spine or restricted by excess hardened connective tissue. Though it is often diagnosed in babies as a congenital condition, tethered cord can remain undetected until adulthood. A rare manifestation of this condition is **occult tethered cord**, and this version does not show on an MRI. Symptoms of tethered cord include back pain, weakness or shooting pains in the legs, problems with control of bowel and/or bladder, tremors in the legs, and visible signs such as high arches and curled toes. If tethered cord is not properly diagnosed and addressed, the long-term outcome can be bleak. Standard of care for tethered cord generally is surgery.

As with many of the rare conditions that can occur with hEDS, a patient will usually be working with an MD and we will not be the ones to identify tethered cord. However, when we have an EDS patient with these symptoms, it helps to know what they are and to be able to communicate with the patient. The patient can then follow up with their MD. It's not that unusual to have EDS patients with tethered cord, just as it is not a tremendous surprise to have a patient who is diagnosed with Chiari. Either at the top of the line or near the bottom, the spinal cord might not be where it should be for optimal health. Awareness of neurological red flags is crucial for those who wish to support EDS populations.

When the fabric is already weakened by connective tissue disorder, there can be a domino effect that seems endless and relentless. And yet, I would take this moment to encourage my colleagues in the profession with the reminder that Chinese medicine is exceptionally useful when it comes to rare and complicated presentations. This chapter has a conclusion. We will move on to more engaging topics.

Before we conclude, in any event, there is more. Rheumatic conditions like **psoriasis**, **ankylosing spondylosis**, and **rheumatoid arthritis** are categorized as autoimmune diseases, not genetic disorders along the lines of the Ehlers-Danlos syndromes. However, these are a collection of soft tissue diseases, and it may come as no surprise that EDS is associated with greater instances of adjacent tissue-related conditions.[13] Psoriasis causes raised, itchy patches on the skin that can be unsightly and debilitating. Lesions commonly appear on the knees, elbows, trunk, and scalp. Ankylosing spondylosis is an inflammatory condition that begins with back or neck pain and may lead to fused areas of the spine. Rheumatoid arthritis causes joint pain, swelling, and decreased range of motion. It usually is bilateral and often affects the smaller joints, such as the fingers and toes. But does the patient also have hypermobile joints? Do they also have soft skin elsewhere, or unusual scars and/or stretch marks? Any time that we see a CTD patient for these conditions, we might consider whether or not the real problem is an HCTD.

People with HCTDs might also have any other autoimmune condition imaginable. Though we are familiar with these conditions, it is helpful to outline them here, with—again—the caveat that we look at the autoimmune signs and then check for HCTD red flags. In my experience, it gets easier and easier to see an autoimmune disease that is just that vs. an autoimmune disease that is nested within an HCTD.

**Lupus**, as we recollect, is an autoimmune disease that presents with extreme fatigue, joint pain, and a butterfly rash across the cheeks. It is a multi-systemic condition that can affect blood, brain, hearts, lungs, skin, and kidneys.

**Sjögren's syndrome** is an autoimmune condition characterized by insufficient moisture production in saliva and tear-producing glands. This disease presents with dry eyes and dry mouth. Women can also suffer from dryness of the vagina. This disease can leave a person with a distorted sense of taste, burning dry eyes and blurred vision, difficulty swallowing, tooth decay, and/or enlarged salivary glands.

**Scleroderma** is an autoimmune disease of too much collagen, leading to thickening of the skin and organs and presenting with patches of hardened skin that are usually found on the trunk of the body. It is not unusual to have an EDS patient who has a relative with scleroderma, and patients with both EDS and Sjögren's syndrome are not unusual. Again, we ask ourselves if it is a matter of the EDS patient having an autoimmune disease or the autoimmune disease patient having EDS. I do not think that anyone knows whether the chicken came first or if it was the egg, but either way, this is painful and challenging for patients.

**Morphea** is a localized and relatively benign form of scleroderma that may also be adjacent to an HCTD patient's presentation. I have seen queries within the hEDS community as to whether there are fellow community members who have some family members with scleroderma and others with hEDS. The answer is yes, and it used to be a little surprising when I first observed such exchanges. Now, with the benefit of experience, I am not surprised. The takeaway? When we have a patient with connective tissue disorder, especially if it is complex, there are often manifestations of something else, something adjacent, in the patient or in their family members.

On this note, I would be remiss if I did not mention **trigger finger (or toe).** Trigger toe is when active plantar flexion causes a toe to lock into position and is a result of stenosing tenosynovitis. This is a relatively unusual condition seen mostly in retired ballerinas. I have treated hEDS patients with it in my clinic. Trigger fingers can happen with anyone, and I have treated EDS patients for this condition as well. As I discuss later, an EDS patient's tendons need special care. The usual protocol of needling tendons in these cases requires particular knowledge when the tendons belong to a body with weak connective tissue.

Softening or hardening of the skin is not the only way that an HCTD patient's body expresses variance. **Raynaud's syndrome** is the temporary disruption of blood flow to the extremities in response to cold or stress. Fingers, toes, ears, and the tip of the nose can all become numb and cold and turn white, blue, or red. In my experience, most EDS patients have either Raynaud's or icy cold feet.[14] Skin that changes color due to sensitivity to external stimuli, rather than to cold, is also extremely common in this patient population. **Dermatographia** is another sensitivity issue, where even lightly scratching on the skin's surface will produce raised welts. Another name for this is skin writing, and it is just what it sounds like. A person can write on their skin just by scraping gently.

Awareness of the possible variations to skin conditions and the immune system will become second nature to a practitioner who routinely treats hEDS patients. When the day comes that we treat our first patient with **MCTD** (also known as **Sharp's syndrome**), we will not be unduly shocked at the notion of multiple autoimmune conditions contained in one single body. It is not a common disease, like **fibromyalgia**, but we can add it to our long list of conditions that are adjacent to, if not part of, the larger picture that includes an HCTD.

For its part, fibromyalgia is highly associated with hEDS and other joint hypermobility syndromes (JHSs). Fibromyalgia is a soft tissue disorder that causes pain throughout the body, fatigue, and sleep problems, and—no surprise, considering—it often causes emotional distress. A patient with hEDS may be diagnosed with both fibromyalgia and hEDS or, as is so unfortunately the case, the patient can be misdiagnosed with fibromyalgia only, leaving the root cause of their pain (hEDS) unattended.[15] Length of time to diagnosis and correct identification of the disease is a factor for many. A patient who is dismissed with a catch-all diagnosis of fibromyalgia may very well eventually learn that the root cause of their suffering is hEDS. We help our patients immeasurably by knowing this and by being able to help them identify their varying signs and symptoms in a way that they can present clearly to their MD if they so choose.

**Anxiety**, **depression**, and/or **grief** may characterize a patient's experience. It stands to reason that chronic pain can set one on the path to depression or anxiety. The sense of destabilized connection and constantly shifting center of gravity when one's body does not hold together in a stable way can cause the same. Being unable to fulfill one's dearest dreams because one is unable to stand for long periods or lift things or otherwise complete required job tasks means losing out on certain careers, not having children for fear of passing along a genetic disease or due to not being able to carry a child without undue harm to one's body, and/or coming to terms with a lifelong disability that may progress may well precipitate a mourning period that has no end or boundaries, and what then? Depression, anxiety, and grief have a different tone and feel when one's own being is the foundation of these emotions. Conversely, what the patient experiences might not even be an issue stemming from the emotions. As I will discuss in forthcoming chapters, dysautonomia's effects can present in ways that are diagnosed as psycho-emotional disorders when, in truth, the root cause is a misfiring autonomic nervous system rather than a trauma response.

**Medical PTSD** is not uncommon, and one framework for assessing it within the EDS community is via the outline provided by the acronym BITTEN.[16] Institutional betrayal is not rare for people with so-called rare diseases. A patient with complex presentations that do not lend themselves well to diagnosis is at the mercy of siloed healthcare systems and overworked practitioners who are unable to spend the proper amount of time with him or her or them.

**Neuro difference** is a category unto itself. People with EDS can be more likely to be either on an **autism spectrum** or diagnosed as **autistic**. This population is also linked to higher incidences of attention deficit hyperactivity disorder (**ADHD**). Whether or not this is a problem, per se, is the patient's decision. Should it be a person's human right to have a pharmaceutical prescription? The way some advocates for early diagnosis and swift treatment argue, it is. On the other hand, my facetious question is then: would it be better if everyone did yoga, drank a spoonful of apple cider vinegar every morning, and tried, say, jade eggs in the yoni or semen retention? I don't know about that, either. There is a happy medium when it comes to neuro difference and ADHD, and our approach to it can start by respectfully listening to the patient. If a patient wants help with their ADHD or other form of neuro difference, they will ask; if they are content as they are, then we can support them in ways that respect and honor their neuro difference. We can boost wellbeing while maintaining proper boundaries and all due acknowledgment for their identities as neurodivergent persons.

Last but not least is the matter of **inflammation** and **toxicity**. When we build a practice that supports HCTD, we often by default treat CTDs. In treating these issues, we find that we also become Lyme literate and well versed in the vagaries of mold sicknesses. **Lyme disease** is caused by four different species of bacteria that are transmitted by tick bite. In Europe and Asia, the common bacteria responsible for Lyme disease are *Borrelia afzelii* and *Borrelia garinii*. In the United States, the honors go to *Borrelia burgdorferi* and *Borrelia mayonii*. The outcome of improperly treated infected can include rash (**erythema migrans**), **joint pain**, and **neurological complications**, including **muscle weakness, Bell's palsy**, and/or **numbness in the limbs**. Longer term complications can include **hepatitis, heart problems**, and **extreme fatigue**. Anyone can get bitten by a tick and experience the catastrophe that is unresolved Lyme disease. A person with an HCTD will likely experience such an event with greater pain, extensive disability, and a longer time to recovery, if recovery is even possible. **Mold illness** can be challenging for anyone, but **mycotoxin** and Lyme in combination can render an EDS patient's life a living hell.

Having read all of this, we understand why a patient might have such an ordeal when it comes to getting diagnosed. In the subsequent section, I address significant issues that a patient will experience on their journey towards identification and categorization. After that, we leave behind (at least for the most part) Western biomedicine and focus, instead, on what we as practitioners of Chinese medicine can do for our patients.

## IV. Diagnosis and Discontent

To diagnose or not to diagnose, that is the question...and a big question it is, indeed. If the variety of presentations constitutes a hydra (and it does), then the matter of identification and categorization represents an obstacle course littered with hurdles and sand traps. This is not the only question, but it is a significant one.[17] Its ramifications extend in both directions, as much towards the patient as to the practitioner. Being diagnosed is to be given a name for one's suffering and it can be tremendously validating. It should, at least in theory, remove doubt. But things often are not clear-cut, even with diagnosis.

Being diagnosed can help a patient in some ways and it can hurt them in others. There can also be a level of grief, fear, and aversion to the newly acquired identity. There are safety concerns and ethical considerations for the practitioner of Chinese medicine that incline us towards a pro-diagnosis stance. Yet many of us came to the practice of Chinese medicine because we are not inclined to march in lockstep with the biomedical industrial complex. Ultimately, the patient needs to decide how they want to understand and categorize their own body; the practitioner, on the other side, must uphold ethical safety standards and remain within their scope of practice. The purpose of the final section of this chapter is to consider the notion of biomedical diagnosis and to outline some ideas regarding what being diagnosed (or not) can mean for patients and for practitioners.

I begin by outlining what kinds of patients we might see in our clinics.

A practitioner of Chinese medicine will probably not see patients with the rare subtypes who are not diagnosed. Even so, it is smart to have an idea of what the variations look like (hence the above list) because HCTDs really are not all that uncommon and they present on a spectrum. Someone with a mild presentation of a subtype that requires biomedical supervision still needs a diagnosis even if they prefer to work with a Chinese medicine practitioner as their primary source of support.

To date, I have treated patients with clEDS. I have had one case where the patient had a milder presentation of aEDS and have seen several with potential kEDS. I know someone socially who has all the signs of pEDS. I have had a number of patients who may have Marfan syndrome. I have treated MCTD and osteogenesis imperfecta. Of the conditions that many of us see in our clinics, I have treated patients with one or more of the following: fibromyalgia, scleroderma, lupus, and Sjögren's syndrome. But the majority of my HCTD patients can be categorized as hypermobile or having hEDS, diagnosed or not.

Not all diagnosed patients are the same and nor are the undiagnosed. Either way, there are particular considerations for us to keep in mind.

We will have patients who are diagnosed and who have a medical team in place. I have had patients whose team included a geneticist, an immunologist, a rheumatologist, a neurologist, a gastroenterologist, a urogynecologist, an orthopedic surgeon, a psychiatrist, a psychotherapist, a nutritionist, a PT, and me, their acupuncturist. Patients on this end of the spectrum generally "get acupuncture" rather than benefit from the full range of Chinese medicine's modalities. The practitioner is a small cog in a large wheel. It helps such patients when we understand their biomedical narrative. The Chinese medicine practitioner can keep an eye out for red flags and can answer questions about how the biomedical side corresponds (or not) with the Chinese medicine side if the patient is interested. Even though Chinese medicine is a small part of that patient's care plan, it is both safer and more affirming to the patient when we understand what they undergo in medical settings other than our own.

In the middle range are patients who have been diagnosed or who are at least aware that they have some form of disorder. These patients are best supported by a practitioner who knows the biomedical narratives. Being able to help a patient to formulate questions to ask their doctor can speed up what might otherwise be a lengthy, disempowering diagnostic journey. Most importantly, it is a matter of safety. Even in the absence of vascular involvement, a person may have comorbidities that require biomedical attention. There are also a number of conditions that present as common complaints but which, if they are housed within a hypermobile body, require a trip to the MD. For example, a patient who has intermittent nausea and extremely lax joints plus easy bruising is experiencing Stomach qi rebellion and the Spleen not controlling the Blood. But we need to keep in mind that they may also have the above-described MALS.

On the other extreme, opposite to the first scenario, is the patient who has no idea that they might have hEDS. One never knows who might want to try acupuncture for pain relief or for intractable allergies or some other comparatively routine issue that is, at root, caused by an HCTD. Maybe this is a patient who suffers mystery illnesses. They have gotten no meaningful support elsewhere so they turn to "alternative medicine" for succor. A knowledgeable practitioner can be of immeasurable worth to such patients. We can support a patient who does not want a diagnosis and monitor them for red flags that would require one. Whichever way the unknowing patient might ultimately decide to proceed, it helps us to help them when we know the landmarks of HCTD. It benefits patients when the practitioner is fluent in the language of biomedicine, particularly when the patient does not know anything about hEDS and we are in a position to educate and support their growing awareness.

Proponents argue that an early diagnosis means that a person will be able to get proper healthcare and become informed about ways to preserve the integrity of their joints for the long term. Whether or not one advocates for diagnosis, it is inarguable that some subtypes require biomedical supervision.

There are patients who do not want a diagnosis. Some patients will be told by their doctors that it is better for them to have an HSD tag in their electronic records because some doctors do not want to treat hEDS patients. Noting the hypermobility without specifying EDS is in the patient's best interests (at least according to their PCP). For others, they do not want anything to do with the systems in place for categorizing and treating hEDS. If an individual does not need to be diagnosed for the sake of safety, it is, I think, their own choice to make. By working within the laws of scope of practice and by keeping patient safety at the forefront, it is certainly possible to provide safe, meaningful care to a person who wants to avoid diagnosis.

Once we begin to work with hEDS on a regular basis, it starts to feel like everyone has some variation or other of an HCTD. However, a practitioner of Chinese medicine is not likely to see an undiagnosed Loeys-Dietz patient, for instance, nor osteogenesis imperfecta, because these are usually distinctive and disabling enough that someone will have flagged the patient within the biomedical system. Marfan syndrome, on the other hand, might not be as readily diagnosed and it is entirely possible to have patients with red flags that point to this condition.[18]

A brief digression on the topic of Marfan syndrome is instructive. How many of us have had patients who are tall, slender, and lanky? This would be a patient with long arms and legs, and maybe they come to our office because they struggle with anxiety or asthma or weak digestion. They just do not feel so good. We notice that they have a dip in their chest or the chest wall protrudes. They may have flat feet, stretch marks across their upper back and rib cage, a slight curve to the spine that we notice upon palpation, and long fingers that reach past their GB-31 point. Marfan syndrome is caused by a gene mutation and it can express as life-threatening or mild. An observant Chinese medicine practitioner will take note of the patient's physiology and chief complaints and take extra care. These are patients who may need to be screened by a geneticist. If the genetic mutation is identified, the patient will need to work with a cardiologist because aortic dissection or rupture is a potential outcome of this condition.

Awareness of EDS has increased exponentially in recent years. Partially, this is due to advances in genetic research. Social media, popular culture, and celebrities with the condition enhance awareness. Sheer numbers of people who are affected by environmental injury on top of whatever genetic foundation underlying their presentation make it harder and harder to ignore histamine intolerance, MCAS, and connective tissue disorder, be it autoimmune or genetic. I predict that hEDS will be a familiar concept to the general public, similar to diabetes, within ten years. So will MCAS and histamine intolerance. These are conditions that are going to increase, not decrease.

Chinese medicine is an excellent recourse for patients who struggle with chronic pain. We can alleviate digestive difficulty regardless of the why. Any time there is a chronic problem, Chinese medicine is an excellent option. Patients who cannot metabolize pharmaceutical drugs the way they are supposed to be metabolized can find support in herbal formulas. So—long story short—there is no end to what Chinese medicine can do for HCTD patients. Having a broad idea of what can be the concerns of an EDS patient and being able to identify, educate, and support patient wellbeing is a pillar of a Chinese medicine practitioner's value to this community. Meeting patients where they are can change a person's life. Knowing what it is, what the common comorbid conditions are, and how to place ourselves and our patient on a spectrum are all crucial steps in the process of building an EDS- and HCTD-supportive practice. Once we have done this, we can then get to what really matters.

To wit: treating our patients with Chinese medicine. Not integrative, with the parameters set by biomedicine, but—instead—with Chinese medicine on its own terms.

# CHAPTER 2

# Chinese Medicine

## HOW WE DIAGNOSE

## I. Getting to the Roots of Diagnostic Approaches

In this chapter, I consider how the needs of HCTD patients fit into a Chinese-medicine-focused intake process and how, given the vagaries of the disorder, there are aspects of it that require illness-specific knowledge. At other times, a syndrome-focused lens is most beneficial. But how does a pattern-centered diagnostic approach fit into this picture, especially given that Chinese medicine does not, strictly speaking, have a designation for HCTDs? This aim of this chapter is to clarify a practitioner's diagnostic point of entry. I discuss the initial intake and consider the theme of seeing in Chinese medicine. What we bring to the table combined with the offerings of our patients contains multitudes.

How, then, might we begin?

An initial clinical encounter, no matter the medical tradition, is universal. A person suffers an ailment and wants relief or, perhaps, they seek preventative care. A physician conducts an intake and makes certain determinations. The contours of this visit and subsequent ones are regulated by clear-cut boundaries, including scope-of-practice laws, practitioner abilities, and patient needs. There is a base level of health (and deviation from it) that constitutes a foundation for these encounters. The practitioner's skill level and the patient's willingness to comply will generally, though not always, predict the outcome. Diagnosis is a starting point that precipitates treatment strategy. These parameters are relatively clear.

Such clarity is uncommon with HCTD patients in any medical context. We as practitioners of Chinese medicine remain aware that scope-of-practice constraints and patient-safety concerns require additional attention when treating complicated disorders that are not entirely well managed by Western medicine. We also do not directly access resources that patients may need, from biotechnology to surgery and other allopathic interventions. This does not in any way, shape, or form suggest that our traditions are of lesser value to a suffering patient.[1] In a multi-systemic hydra like EDS, diagnosis becomes a shifting metaphor. The way Chinese medicine builds a case for interpretation of sign and symptom is, in my experience, ideally suited for the exigencies of complex disorders like hEDS.

But what do we mean by the term "diagnosis"?

Nigel Ching's excellent resource, *The Art and Practice of Diagnosis in Chinese Medicine,* outlines the avenues that a practitioner might follow when parsing signs and symptoms. *Bian bing lun zhi* (differentiation of symptoms and signs in relation to disease category), he explains, privileges Western biomedicine, while *bian zheng lun zhi* (differentiation of signs and symptoms in relation to imbalance) relies on a traditional perspective that values pattern identification (2017, p.17). In a way, the *bian zheng* approach has become collateral damage to the forces of contemporary medicine. Karchmer's fieldwork as a student in Beijing highlights what is, in essence, an existential crisis of contemporary practice. Viewing Chinese medicine through a postcolonial lens, he ruefully notes that practitioners have, to a certain degree, lost confidence in their traditions. The outcome is that, "When the two medical systems are viewed as radically different and the epistemological authority of biomedicine is unquestioned, pattern discrimination becomes an impoverished version of disease diagnosis. Chinese medicine becomes useful only when one approaches the therapeutic limits of Western medicine" (2022, p.184). This is an attitude we see outside of China as well, unfortunately.

Privileging one diagnostic language over the other is not an academic debate. When we specialize in chronic illnesses that elude Western biomedicine's attempts to define, contain, and resolve them, we are better able to serve our patients by becoming bilingual critical thinkers. It is a thorny issue, one that encompasses not only patient care but also ways of thinking, modes of practice, and development of professional identity. When we choose one and the other, we take part in the construction of meaning in Chinese medicine. We build, as a result, a lived practice in the way that border communities build lived cultures and languages that are neither one nor the other, but a combination of both.

The more adept we become, the more knowledgeably creative we can be; this, ultimately, benefits a patient population that needs, above all, options. One diagnosis and one protocol may "work" for some patients but it does not for most of them. Not when we're dealing with HCTDs plus comorbidities.

Online communities offer ways for us to continue learning. Ching, when in these milieux, notes that he sees the question, "Which acupuncture points should you use to treat some Western named disorder?" and explains that he disagrees with this for three reasons. By relying on rote treatments of Western-framed diseases via acupuncture points in this manner, the practitioner risks predicating treatment on an incorrect diagnosis (Western can be wrong too, he reminds). Further, a diagnosis based on a Western model of pathology that does not necessarily correspond with Chinese understandings of same renders the treatment potentially off-target and thus ineffective. Finally, Ching asserts, doing so forgets that the same disorder can have many causes. We rely on a combination of both methods, but the *bian bing* approach is, according to Ching, a default to Western biomedicine (2017, pp.26–27).

Privileging one lens over the other should be intentional but it can become automatic and unthinking. It is a process of learning and discernment to create a language of diagnosis. Some realms where Chinese medicine has found great success do rely on skill with *bian bing* thought process. Consider the work of oncology acupuncturists or those who specialize in fertility. The practitioner's role is clear, and it is hard to argue with the success of an integrative approach. Western medicine has the technology to provide surgeries, radiation, and chemotherapy; Chinese medicine has the techniques and modalities to support healing from their sequelae. Fertility treatments such as IVF originate in the lab and the MD's office; nurturing implantation and a subsequent successful pregnancy is the gift of Chinese medicine's knowledge and practice. In either scenario, it is pragmatic to start from the perspective of *bian bing* and to interpret matters in a Western-leaning way. This is not so with HCTDs, especially not in the context of diagnosis.

Volker Scheid, in outlining the role of Chinese medicine in contemporary China, states that, "Patients treated in Chinese medicine clinics...tend to suffer from chronic diseases or from problems that have not responded to biomedical care" (2002, p.108). We see this outside of China too. Yet even when geneticists single out an offending mutation, an EDS patient will present with comorbidities that defy the authority conferred by the genetic marker. Some of our patients will come to Chinese medicine already diagnosed by Western medicine but will be unable to find meaningful biomedical healthcare even though they have been diagnosed therein. Does the practitioner help this patient by matching presentation with a disease category that is defined by Western medicine (*bian bing*) in these instances? Or does it foster greater critical thinking (and thus more astute detective skills) to rely on the precepts of *bian zheng* and look for syndromes, interrelationships, and imbalance?

The interpretation of Chinese doctors can guide a modern-day practitioner. We are reminded that:

> Bian zheng lunzhi can be divided into two stages. In pattern discrimination, the information, symptoms, and signs collected through the Four Examinations (sizhen) (looking, listening/smelling, asking, and palpation) are analyzed and synthesized to determine the cause, type, location, and relative strength of the pathogen and patient's own constitution (xiezheng guanxi). This culminates in the discrimination of a pattern. In treatment determination, a treatment principle is determined according to the results of pattern discrimination. (Wu Dunxu, Liu Yanchi, and Li Dexin quoted in Karchmer 2022, p.164)

Developing a facility for this is not as easy as memorizing clichéd declarations about Liver overacting on Spleen or being able to recite the signs of Heart–Kidney disharmony. Karchmer provides an overview of textbook history in China and notes, "the pattern-centered modality turns on having a recognized and standardized catalog of the most common patterns" (*ibid.*, p.165). Chinese students, he explains, rely on textbooks that are constrained by political and ideological strictures.[2] Given my experience in American academia, I can say without hesitation that students in this country face identical obstacles.

An added barrier for those of us who do not speak the language consists of cultural and linguistic gatekeepers. There is a vast body of extant medical and historical literature, but who decides what is worthy of translation? Once chosen, and once translated, the text becomes part of the public imaginaries found in academic and clinical discourses. This is all well and good, but readers are still at the mercy of the translator's skill and will remain so unless they learn the target language, which, in the case of classical Chinese, can be out of reach for many.

At the time of this writing, there is a growing corpus of excellent translations. It is also true that some of what we now have is out of date. Certainly, the very existence of the translation contributes to knowledge but when it is erroneous or outdated, then what? Do anthropologists and medical historians provide worthy guidance as we build our home libraries? My answer to that is to say yes...and no. I read the world the way a comparative literature scholar does: interpretation is the result of comparison. As a licensed practitioner, I read certain resources produced by anthropology, psychology, history, and varying humanities fields and recognize that I would have loved them and found them marvelous when I was a Spanish professor. Now, as a practitioner, I think they are nice for sparking critical thought and some, to damn with faint praise, are interesting. But they do not help me to become a better clinician. On the other hand, nor would relying only on science books.[3]

Things would be different if I were a fluent speaker of Mandarin and an accomplished reader of classical Chinese. There are many of us who will say the same thing: *oh, if only...* knowing very well that we have neither the time nor the energy to dedicate to language acquisition.[4]

How, then, do we build our critical thinking skills? And how might we apply them to complex conditions? In our search for authenticity, we might return to claims of such legitimacy within the dichotomy of *bian zheng* against *bian bing*. We might also recognize that, as Karchmer argues, "The claim that *bianzheng lunzi* is the 'essence' of Chinese medicine is perhaps not historically accurate, but it does indeed capture its paramount significance to contemporary practice" (*ibid.*, p.215). As a practitioner who works with complex illness, questions regarding which diagnostic method to privilege do pull at me and they should as well tug at anyone who seeks to develop agile critical thinking skills in the clinical space. For me, the *bian zheng* approach offers an opportunity to practice building my theoretical foundation in a comparative way. It is more challenging than to simply rely on a disease-oriented investigation. I have to try harder, and that's a good thing when one engages with complex conditions.

How we might acquire fluency in this realm of Chinese medicine is not so different than how we would do so in the study of literature and languages not our own. It is, to a certain degree, similar to my early years of graduate school in my first program. Chinese medicine privileges lineage, so I will be forgiven for mentioning that I come from an academic family. My mother, a noted scholar in her own right, advised me to find theorists whose work I admired and to read them specifically to learn to think and communicate at their levels. As a graduate student in my first program, I spent countless hours reading critical analysis and theory and copying out by hand the passages I admired. This is not the same as making flash cards (I made a lot of flash cards in the second graduate program). The time it takes to hand-copy dense theoretical meanderings is the time required to actually imbibe such modes of thinking. As a practitioner now, I have returned to this mode of learning.

This is hard work and it requires dedication. However, if we wish to meaningfully treat complex illness with mindfully delivered Chinese medicine, then we must read a vast range of seminal texts and we do need to constantly and intentionally practice *bian zheng* diagnostics. As we move from one to the other and back again, we want to be aware that we are doing so and focus on what we are learning from each. I very much agree with Liu Lihong when he states that, "Serious study of the classics is able to stretch the limits of our understanding, to broaden our perspective" (2019, p.55). He is correct. Dante's *Commedia* becomes easier and easier to comprehend upon review, and so does the *Shang Han Lun* or the *Nei Jing*. According to Dr. Liu, "The content of the classics are just like this. Before one has uncovered them, they are extremely mysterious. Afterward, they seem very simple" (*ibid.*, p.57).

This does not mean that we are compelled to read these texts for clinical knowledge. Some of us aspire to become scholar-physicians of classical Chinese medicine, others are perfectly satisfied with a traditional Chinese medicine (TCM) approach. There is room for all of us, but we are better thinkers in our traditions when we know our classical sources well and can engage with the languages of them, even if it is only in translation.

Yanhua Zhang's commentary on reading the classics in order to develop intellectual agility is instructive. As she notes, "*Lilun* (theory) in Chinese medicine is rather a discussion of and a reasoning out of the concrete and complicated relations among all the factors relevant to a particular illness course and manipulating the particular relations to effect a cure" (2007, p.25). It is not, today, a way of identifying one correct answer or a source of clinical wisdom in the form of textbook standards of care. Instead, reading and rereading becomes a process of intellectual acculturation. It is a building of ways to think, in that, "The process of learning medical classics is then a process of familiarizing oneself with the way, the style, and the language by which a particular exemplary physician demonstrated his art of medicine" (*ibid.*, p.26).

We must be prepared to study not just primary but also secondary and tertiary resources from a variety of disciplines. What anthropology has to say about Chinese medicine can help us to meaningfully read Chinese medical classics on one hand and our patients' signs and symptoms on the other. So can illness memoirs written by people who have minimal understanding of our medical traditions, as I argue in chapter six. When I specialized in national trauma in my first career, I did not only focus solely on the cause and effect of profound suffering. Rather, I circled around the fulcrum (the trauma itself) and added meaning by considering a multitude of factors, including the legal, medical, and historical. We do the same when we are trying to overcome cultural and linguistic barriers. We do the same when attempting to decipher the many threads that, pulled together, constitute hEDS.

Ching speaks of the seasoned practitioner as being intuitive. This is not, he asserts, an unthinking reflex or a gut-sense intuition. Instead, it is a response that comes from substantive knowledge of a norm (patient population and what health or lack in this population is) and the language of syndromes and patterns (*bian zheng*). In the context of HCTDs, knowing what that norm encompasses requires considerable experience treating different bodies. If we are a member of this patient population, this does not automatically confer knowledge.[5] The only way to become proficient in the norms of HCTD is to practice and to place one's diagnosing fingertips on a range of bodies. Until one is genuinely experienced, it is safer and more productive to rely on the language of *bian bing*. This is especially true if a patient comes to the clinical encounter with a Western biomedical diagnosis in hand. Patients also understand the treatment strategy if it is framed within a Western-leaning outline, which is useful.

Once a practitioner is in possession of substantive experience, the choice of lens can switch. This is not to advocate for a complete negation of Western biomedicine's terms, views, and definitions. Instead, it is an effort to encourage the use of wide-ranging thought processes for the benefit of the patient. We can all agree that Chinese medicine is exceptionally valuable for hard-to-treat chronic illnesses. The *bian zheng* lens allows us to look at these complex cases with an expansive perspective even if we ultimately articulate matters in languages nearer to our own, assuming this "we" is not native Chinese and/or adept at reading classical Chinese medical texts. As Ching points out, "Western medicine trains practitioners to distinguish symptoms separately and to understand them individually or as part of a particular disease or disorder. In Chinese medicine, it is the opposite. Here one is trained to try to see patterns in the symptoms and signs and to see how these are related and what they can be an expression of" (2017, p.19).

When we follow this thought process, and routinely ask

ourselves why we chose one or the other, we develop the agility of thought that we need in order to treat HCTDs. Ultimately, we are able to achieve a more comprehensive benefit for the patient.[6]

Opting for one before the other is a philosophical choice. However, in the case of complex disease, there are tangible reasons in favor of one vs. the other. In part, this section is an argument for *bian zheng lun zhi*, although perhaps my circumlocutions imply otherwise. In relating the way Dr. Sun, one of Karchmer's professors at the University of Beijing, approached and resolved a case, we are given to understand the physician's affirmation that Chinese medicine does not seek to find one answer. Rather, he avows, there are always, "different paths, different points of attacks, different methods, including diametrically opposed methods for curing an illness," and the way to achieve one's desired outcome is to, "seize hold of a single thread, to stick to one theory [and to see it through]" (2022, p.228). To this, I will say *yes, absolutely!* However, I say so with a caveat, and it is that we who do not speak the language need to sift through threads wrought not only by the Chinese medical texts nor simply via biomedical research but, instead, by a wide range of resources.

My argument is for mindful, systematic practice of *bian zheng*. We need to know the Western biomedical narrative and can either stop there or we can translate the concepts into *bian bing*. This is for safety and scope of practice. But for critical thinking and the sort of creativity that leads to better patient outcomes when dealing with complex conditions, we are much more successful when we are fluent in a multicultural expression of *bian zheng*. This takes practice, consistency, the willingness to explore, and the ability to view and review the way we synthesize what is often conflicting information.

But once again, I am getting ahead of myself.

The focus of this chapter is, in essence, pragmatic. In the following section, I provide a model of the initial intake with guidelines on how to filter all of these considerations through the lens of HCTD, setting aside, at least for the moment, digressions regarding critical thought and knowledge acquisition.

How might we find our thread and seize hold of it?

# II. The Four Diagnostic Methods

Taking recourse in the wisdom of Dr. Liu, I argue for the value of traditional diagnostic methods by sharing a quote from *Classical Chinese Medicine*. I felt affirmed when I read his declaration that, "Modern diagnostic tests are no substitute for the four methods of TCM diagnosis: looking, smelling, questioning, and palpating" and saddened by his subsequent admonition that, "Nevertheless, the application of these methods is rapidly declining and the practice of Chinese medicine languishes" (2019, p.233). Based on my clinical experience, I believe that there is no substitute for the four diagnostic methods. However, in the instance of HCTD, we are most successful if we adjust our lens in order to accommodate the languages of dysfunctional connective tissue.

## Observation

Recourse to biomedical screening methods does not confer an advantage in the clinical realm. A practitioner who is familiar with EDS presentations can and will read the body visually and can and will come to meaningful conclusions regarding syndromes, patterns, and healing modalities even without advanced diagnostic technologies. EDS patients are members of a population that tends to suffer medical gaslighting and they often require inordinate lengths of time before diagnosis. A practitioner who simply pays attention is worth their weight in gold. Do we not all want to feel seen? There is an intangible, emotional quality to seeing and being seen; in the clinical encounter, creating the sense for the patient that the practitioner looks, and sees, can begin a healing process.[7]

What do we look for when we make use of the diagnostic pillar that is observation?

When greeting a new patient, we take note of the complexion. What does the skin look like? When we have worked with enough EDS patients, it becomes possible to spot difference in skin quality even in photographs. The patient's outer wrapper, their skin, is an important clue. In cases related to collagen and connective tissue, this is a primary source of information. Relative to people who do not have EDS, their skin will more likely than not have a porcelain quality to it that will be easily noted by an experienced clinician.

Smooth skin, though seemingly enviable, is generally accompanied by other, less-felicitous signs. Flat, papery scars are another allusion to collagen disorder, as are stretch marks, especially when they are on areas that might not normally be covered by such lesions. Some patients will have ribs and paraspinal areas that are marked with flat, shiny, wide stretch marks. Others will have atrophic scars that are fine and crinkled like cigarette paper and, if the person is Black or naturally more dark-skinned, the tissue might be a lighter hue than one would normally see in a scar on a person with abundant melatonin. Collagen that does not function properly does not create robust scars. Stretch marks on a body with connective tissue disorder do not present the way they do on a sturdier dermis.

How the patient walks can speak volumes. Observing how their body moves in space and against its own joints is instructive. Though biomedicine does not know precisely why people with EDS tend to have sensory dysfunction, including lack of balance, one theory is that lax joints and weaker tissues do not communicate well to and from the brain. Whatever the cause, a practitioner should not be surprised by ungainliness. If the patient is not clumsy, perhaps they walk in such a way that there is obvious pain in the joints. With or without impaired proprioception, a person with EDS will often bruise easily. This is due not to trauma but, instead, to weakness and instability of the vessels as part of their collagen dysfunction. Petechiae on random areas of the body are not uncommon.

Complexion and visible bruises and movement patterns are easy to see even before the patient sits down. Once seated, a practitioner might notice that the patient winds their feet around the legs of the chair in ways that a stiffer person would never be able to do.[8] If the practitioner observes the patient holding a pen while finalizing paperwork at the initial intake, it can be telling if their fingers bend backwards at the proximal and/or distal interphalangeal joints. If the fingers are hypermobile, a practitioner can ask the patient to extend the metacarpal joints in what is called a "flying bird hand sign." Not everyone can bend their fingers backwards so that their hand looks like the wings of a bird; this is indicative of hypermobility.

Joints that exceed normal range of extension might include elbows and knees that extend further than what might be expected. The patient, if already diagnosed, might mention their number on the Beighton scale. This test is named after Peter Beighton, a geneticist and an early pioneer of Ehlers-Danlos classification, and it is part of a biomedical diagnostic process. Though a Chinese medicine practitioner will not use the Beighton scale to diagnose patients (we do not diagnose EDS, and it is not necessarily appropriate to make use of the Beighton scale in this context), the patient may know their number and want it to be included in their chart.[9]

Feet can communicate volumes. Does the patient have flat feet? Are there small bumps on the heels? Piezogenic papules, or visible little fatty nodules, are the result of weak connective tissue that is unable to hold fat in a stable position. A patient may have excess ossification laid across the navicular bone and tenderness or bruising or other signs of dysfunction along with it.

This condition, called accessory navicular syndrome, can cause pain, inflammation, and increased instability in the ankle and up to the knee. "Do you have extra bone across that bump on the inside of your foot?" is a relatively common question on social media EDS support groups; often, individuals will report having this presentation in one foot and not the other. An unstable foot or feet is common in EDS.

Visual clues abound. As we build practices that specifically address connective tissue disorder, we begin to notice signs and symptoms of hypermobility almost everywhere we look. At some point or another, a practitioner will see clues even where they are not necessarily indicative of the condition. This, too, shall pass. The more extensive the experience, the more readily we are able to deem a sign or symptom useful...or not. Some people just are more flexible than others and it's not clinically significant. Other people are stiff, especially if they are over the age of thirty or so, but that does not mean that they are not members of the hEDS community. Tight muscles may be holding lax joints as stable as possible for their body but the joints are no less unstable and the patient is probably in just as much pain as they would be otherwise. It's a different sort of pain, but it is disabling nonetheless.

With EDS, a clinician is generally going to be able to identify more than one syndrome pattern, and often, they will contradict each other. Learning the basic visuals makes the ensuing multiplicity much more comprehensible.

## Listening and Smelling

"When you hear hoofbeats, think of horses not zebras" is an aphorism coined in the 1940s by Dr. Theodore Woodward, a professor at the University of Maryland School of Medicine. This is taught to medical students as a way of reminding them to think of the common and everyday diagnosis rather than the unique or rare one. The zebra is the mascot of the Ehlers-Danlos community because hoofbeats can and do mean zebras—or rarity—when it comes to this condition.[10] One will not, at least one hopes not, hear hoofbeats in our clinics. Regardless, EDS patients do not tend to have a distinctive sound profile that differs from what one might hear from any other patient.

And yet, there are exceptions.

Does the patient's jaw click? When they move, is there audible crepitus issuing from their joints? Such noises, coupled with a greenish tinge around the mouth, are a clue. What can we notice about their vocal tone? Any subtype of EDS can affect the throat and vocal cords, leading to difficulty in swallowing, speaking, and breathing easily. In such patients, we can hear the effects of this presentation.

Smell can be instructive, depending on the range of symptoms the patient brings to the clinical space. Not all scents can be directly attributed to EDS. The sweetish smell indicative of diabetes can be detected on anyone with this metabolic disorder; it isn't a clue for EDS. Yet smell is part of a larger picture, so noticing odor and being able to discern where it fits and whether it is relevant to EDS is a skill to cultivate. I had, for example, a patient who not only was diagnosed with EDS but also had multiple other conditions, including kidney disease. A faint odor of bleach characterized their feet and it ebbed and flowed in pungency as their disease progressed.

A note on smells must also include a reminder that the practitioner learns quite a bit from smelling, but using one's nose goes both ways. A patient may be (as so many patients in an acupuncture clinic are) sensitive to smells. If a practitioner expects to see a good number of hEDS patients, they need to implement a "no-perfume" policy in their clinic. Scented soaps, any perfumes, and—unfortunately—moxibustion can result in extreme responses in EDS patients, especially if they also present with MCAS. By this, I do not mean a headache or nausea. Some people can have an anaphylactic response to the smell of burning herbs.[11] A practitioner who wishes to work with HCTD patients will choose one or the other but it is not safe to have a clinic that treats HCTDs and offers moxibustion.

## Palpation

When we think of palpation, we may think only of the pulse and perhaps what we do when we look for tender spots. However, the ability to read the body via touch is crucial for a practitioner who works with HCTD patients. Developing this skill requires practice, dedication, and experience. Many of us are not taught channel theory or exceptional palpation skills and this is lamented by practitioner-scholars who know the genuine value of this diagnostic pillar. In my estimation, palpation is one of our best, if not the most efficacious, diagnostic gifts.

I learned about EDS by my sense of touch. In student clinic, I attracted patients with joint problems and chronic pain. As I practiced finding tender spots, I marveled at the feel of these bodies. I know what my own body feels like. As someone who essentially grew up in the gym and whose early years were formed by proximity to bodybuilding culture, my loose joint connections and hyperflexibility drew comment. But so did my capacity to easily put on muscle. My tendons were stretchy but they were solid. My intimate relationships were unremarkable in this regard as well. Bodies, at least as I knew them before student clinic, were fairly muscular and I never noticed tendons. If I was always the bendy one in my relationships, it was unremarkable given that women tend to be more flexible than men anyway.

Before student clinic, I had never touched a body with tendons like cornsilk. Before student clinic, I didn't know that some people's skin could stretch like water. Before student clinic, I didn't know anything about the Ehlers-Danlos syndromes, and what I learned, I really did learn by palpating.

Palpating hyperflexible bodies sent me straight to my books.

I did remember the picture in my biology textbook of the contortionist. There I found the term "Ehlers-Danlos syndrome" and knew I was onto something. I kept studying. I kept palpating. I joined together puzzle pieces that included my own experiences with a knee that repeatedly subluxed, a hip joint that came entirely out of the socket when I stretched too far one day, and my double-jointed fingers that bent backwards more than anyone else I had ever met. When a clinician palpates with listening fingers and hands that see, they learn. Maybe the practitioner learns things about their own self, as I did, but certainly we learn about patients and their bodies' stories.

An hEDS body may have multiple joints with tendons and ligaments that feel like cornsilk: fine, thin, slippery, and breakable. Most patients that I have treated tend to have only one or two joints like this, while the rest of the skeleton is held together with connections that feel like embroidery thread or yarn. The cornsilk joint will be the one that has subluxed repeatedly. Other patients do not feel this way at all, but maybe they have a sensation of smoothness and water where fascia would generally be dense and textured. Patients like this tend to be colder and may have the blue fingers associated with Raynaud's disease. There is often a slippery quality to the skin, as though its connection to the tensile fabric beneath it were tenuous and unreliable.

The palpation of an EDS body must be gentle. The patient will, almost always, be in pain. One does not wish to begin the therapeutic connection by inflicting more on the patient. Also, we learn more by being diplomatic in asking the body to speak. A lifelong need to guard joints means that the tissues will reject anything that comes at them aggressively. This includes palpating fingers. If the practitioner gets anything, they get an "Ouch" and resistance if they are not gentle. But they will not gain the information that we need. Plus, one could injure a patient by pushing or pulling with too much force. One of my patients had an unstable atlantooccipital joint and was at risk if they sneezed too hard. Another booked a massage while on vacation. The therapist did not listen when my patient asked her to be careful and she tore a muscle in my patient's hip as a result.[12] Not all hEDS patients are this disabled, but some are, and it is the clinician's job to be mindful of this fact.

My teacher, Dr. Fan, always insisted that students assess a patient by starting on the side that is not injured, painful, or dysfunctional. This is sound advice. When a practitioner knows how "the good knee" is constructed, or what a non-painful part of the body feels like, or what the movement of the tendons over the palm of the less-dysfunctional hand involves, for instance, then palpating its opposite is instructive. If a patient comes for treatment of ankle pain or for carpal tunnel syndrome, we start by assessing "the good side" and then, subsequently, move to the distal joint of the opposite limb or structure. Gently, gently, with listening hands and fingers that see, we move from elbow to wrist or ankle to knee. Does the limb get colder as we approach the fulcrum of the chief complaint? Do we notice a subtle, increased hint of edema or crispiness to the subsurface of the skin? If there are nodules, they will be subtle but, in an EDS body, the subtle cues are the ones that speak volumes. Is it possible to discern changes in texture of skin?

It takes practice to develop confidence when touching patients who might be fragile. Learning the tactile strategies that are effective with hEDS bodies takes time. I spent the first years of my tui na practice working with my eyes shut. Even now, I close my eyes and open them onto my fingertips when I want to truly view a limb or structure. There is a difference, and there are different needs, when a body has a disordered connective tissue. The practitioner must learn to read that body in terms of relative relation between substance (muscle, tendon, bone) and form (ligament to bone; tendon to muscle; one bone to another at the joint). We learn to follow fascial planes readily as we move along the contour of muscle and bone. Everything counts. *Everything*.

Our attitude makes a difference. Are we calm and centered and open to hearing what the patient's body wants to share? Is our jaw relaxed and our facial expression peaceful? What is the difference in size between clinician and patient? If the practitioner is large and the patient small, it is best to sit down when palpating. Looming over anyone is not a good idea anyway, but with patients who are in pain, and those who have had bad experiences at the doctor's office, it is crucial to be aware of body positioning, both that of the practitioner and that of the patient.

I tell patients that we will be chatty during the first treatment so that I can learn how their body tenses up or relaxes while conversing. Like Dr. Wang Ju-Yi in *Applied Channel Theory in Chinese Medicine: Wang Ju-Yi's Lectures on Channel Therapeutics* (hereafter *Applied Channel Theory*), I am a practitioner who holds friendly exchanges to get information from patients, all the while palpating and listening with my fingers just as much as with my ears (2008, p.xxii). In subsequent appointments, the patient is cordially invited to nap during treatment, but in the first, I do want to feel what happens when they speak. This is a valuable investigative tactic.

In effect, we are looking for information, we are developing a relationship of trust, and we share the energy of our hands. For one practitioner, healing is mediated via the acupuncture needle; for another, it is gua sha or cupping or tui na. Either way, contact is through our hands. When working with connective tissue disorder, it is especially important to be mindful of the hands' message. The questions a practitioner might want to consider include: Do I love the human skeleton? Do I feel a sense of awe at the beauty of tendons and fascia and muscle? Am I able to approach the patient's physical self with respect and care? Patients know, on a deep level, what the answers to these questions are and, before touching them, the practitioner should know these answers too. Being mindfully, deliberately respectful in one's approach to another's body should be a factor in our dealings with all patients, if we ponder it, but it is especially significant when we aspire to work with connective tissue disorder.

Another reason to tread lightly is the matter of medical PTSD. Though this is a topic I address in a later chapter, its relevance to the matter of palpation is inarguable. People with EDS can spend a decade or more trying to find out why they are in such pain or how it is that they have unrelenting GI problems. They do not know why their immune system reacts violently to mundane triggers. Some pass out when they stand up and nobody figures out why. If they go to a PT, maybe the PT exacerbates their issues. Maybe they went to another acupuncturist who was an utter clod. The MD dismissed them by saying that they needed to lose weight or said that things were due to anxiety. Possibly, our brand-new patient has been poked and prodded and gaslit to the point of utter desperation. One never knows and it is better not to find out by causing further pain. Patients who have been wounded elsewhere can be fearful. People who have been seen by multiple practitioners may have deep psychic wounds that leave them vulnerable.

Someone who has been endlessly examined and prodded might, like a humble and docile beast of burden, quietly submit to being palpated yet one more time. But it hurts them to do so. It suggests to them that their body is not their own, and nobody needs that. Especially not our chronic illness folks. When we palpate our hEDS patients, we absolutely must take into account the way their tissue is constructed. It is tissue that injures easily. We also must take into consideration their emotional landscape and need for dignity and boundaries. Their souls can injure easily too.

Some of the things that patients have told me about being touched and tested and screened and assessed are heartbreaking. Though there may not be any intent to invade their dignity, the aphorism attributed to Bion of Borysthenes is also true: the boys throw stones at the frogs in jest, but the frogs die in earnest.

Intention does not always transfer to outcome. In my clinic, I teach patients about consent. My patients are encouraged to assert their boundaries when they feel like it, so they know that if one day, one area is permissible and the next time, not, that is just fine by me. I think that all patients need to learn that their consent is a key aspect of treatment. But our chronic pain patients need it most of all, especially when their pain is caused by orphan diseases or medical mysteries that have sent them to a long string of medical appointments that came up with little or no useful information.

I ask permission before touching. We are a team, the hEDS patient and me, and we negotiate location and palpation depth. When we do this, we encourage patients to develop confidence in their interactions with other healthcare practitioners. It also alleviates any fear of being injured. We need to ask them questions that speak to the way they experience their bodies, too. A body in pain will always respond affirmatively to the question, "Is this a tender spot?" A better question is, "How does this feel?" We will remember that some people with hEDS bruise very easily.

Palpation is the very best and most informative diagnostic tool we have when working with an EDS patient. Our ability to read the body via touch will inform what modalities we can offer. A clinician who wants to work with HCTD patients absolutely must learn a register of touch that responds directly to the needs of this patient population. It is a specific one. There is a learning curve for it. Thus, we practice, we put in the time, and we learn from each and every patient with EDS who comes in our door.

Both practitioner and patient benefit from dedication to learning the art of palpation.

## Interview

A jewel in the crown of Chinese medicine is the initial intake. With EDS patients, there are added layers to this process and our capacity to listen is fundamental. Dr. Liu reminds that, "Those with clinical experience know that there are patients with very complicated conditions. … They speak at length, but there is inevitably a sentence, or a symptom, or a pulse that arouses your attention, and it is this that will lead you to their primary symptoms" (2019, p.170). Finding our thread with HCTD patients requires a broad understanding not just of medical theory but also of human nature. We need to be good listeners. The initial interview contains multitudes.

First and foremost, this is an opportunity to establish trust. Not all EDS patients are traumatized. However, enough of them are that we move slowly and make certain to demonstrate active listening skills. Some initial appointments will consist almost solely of speaking and listening. If one has never worked with an EDS patient who has MCAS and POTS, plus a long list of other seemingly random ailments, then it might be surprising how long it takes to complete a patient history.[13] And yet, we want our patients to feel heard.

It helps to acknowledge that there is a lot to say, and it may take more than one visit to get the whole story. A seasoned patient will know the drill and be comfortable. An anxious patient might differ. Meghan O'Rourke's poignant assertion resonates, "In the absence of certainty, medical science remains unsure what story to tell. Too often it turns away from patients rather than listening to the long and chaotic stories we tell, narratives that start and stop and double back, searching for meaning in the peculiar rash that broke out that day or the car accident that triggered pain or the death after which nothing was the same" (2022, p.229). Knowing how profoundly important it is for the patient to be able to speak and be heard, we might focus on the broader picture and maybe on one specific issue, but we reassure the patient that we want to hear them and we are willing to listen.

Listening is not just a matter of relationship building. It also entails practical components that help us to conduct a safer visit.

Whether or not the patient has been diagnosed, a tendency towards vertigo is something to know before moving to the treatment table, for example. One of my patients once told me a heartbreaking story about going to the doctor and being scolded because they couldn't get up off the examination table quickly. The assistant said, "It must be nice to be able to lay around all day" and tried to hustle my patient along. A person who suffers from POTS is not going to move off the table simply because the practitioner is aggressive. Instead, they might faint and hit their head against the floor. Factoring this in before the first treatment is much safer for the patient and certainly less stressful for the practitioner. It should be routine to ask about syncope and vertigo when working with hEDS patients.

Dysautonomia is a common comorbidity. Does the patient have slow digestion and a history of constipation? What about their temperature? Do they break into spontaneous sweat without any apparent reason? What about anxiety? A dysregulated nervous system produces many, many health challenges. Being able to separate what is caused by faulty collagen and what is exacerbated by mixed nervous system signals means the difference between strategic treatments that genuinely help a patient or, instead, ones that do little other than mindlessly react to surprises when they occur. Parsing dysautonomia requires diplomacy and a good listening ear. Being patient, listening carefully, and being ready to hear the same story more than once is the only way to decipher the vagaries of a dysregulated autonomic nervous system.

Some people start out their lives with not a whisper of symptoms or signs. After having a concussion, everything changes and suddenly, they have full-blown EDS. Other patients will be part of a large family history that has always shown evidence of this condition. There is some question about EDS being mediated by mast cell disorder. EDS is multi-systemic, it is variable, and it is unique to each and every patient.

The intake interview needs to take all of this into account.

If a practitioner follows the ten-questions format, it is useful to know that the ten questions require an EDS filter for greatest efficacy. How I ask them and what I listen for when hearing the response depends on whether my patient is diagnosed or not. Sometimes, I'll ask the questions and, in getting the answer, I'll start to piece together a diagnostic map that includes potential HCTD. It all depends. But there are specific things to keep in mind if one intends to address the concerns of HCTD patients.

The ten questions, in order, are:

## Hot or Cold?

The patient will often be cold. Hands and feet especially, but frigid regions can also include the low back or abdomen. As a practitioner in Texas, where summer heat can often go over a hundred degrees, my EDS patients will still ask to have the heat lamp on their feet when outside it is stunningly hot. What can be useful is to notice where on any given channel the body is cooler. For example, I have had patients whose legs are icy right where the Spleen and the Liver channels exchange relative pathways. Focusing on Cold yields valuable information that will help the practitioner to make a meaningful syndrome identification and treatment strategy.

Since Cold is the norm, it is telling if there is Heat anywhere. A patient with MCAS can present with extremes of Wind and Heat (wheals, hives). An hEDS patient who is normally freezing may present with yin deficiency Heat that comes and goes. Heat in the Blood and the Spleen not controlling the vessels can lead to petechiae.

## Sweating

It is typical to find that a patient either experiences spontaneous sweating, hands and feet perspiration, and/or the typical sign of yin deficiency that is demonstrated by night sweats. Some patients do not sweat at all and instead experience edema in their fingers and toes.

## Regarding the Head and Face

Migraine history is fairly common with this population, as are eye floaters, tinnitus, and vertigo. A practitioner should not be surprised to hear that the patient experiences internal Wind, leading to facial numbness or Bell's palsy. Intermittent flushing of the skin or the bright red cheeks of yin deficient Heat are not unusual. The patient might have slightly blue sclera (or very blue sclera). It is not unusual to see a faint green ring around the mouth or subtle smudge of black under the eyes that alludes to the Kidneys.

If we are concerned, it is useful to remember that vEDS can show in the facial features.[14]

## Pain

Pain is an individualized experience for each one of us. With EDS, perception of pain is altered. When a person lives with pain each and every day, they adjust to it. Normal pain for an hEDS body is unimaginable torture to someone who knows little about chronic pain. Asking an EDS patient to rate their pain on a 1–10 scale may not garner meaningful information. Learning to hear how a patient describes their experience gives us keys and tools. How does the patient narrate their experience?

Pain in an hEDS body can be traced to a joint that has sub-luxed repeatedly. Pain can suffuse the entire body, leaving the person exhausted and overly sensitive to all stimuli. Pain can be referred or it begins and ends in one place. Pain can depend on the rhythms of the Chinese organ clock. Pain may be confined to certain joints, as though it resided in the bones. It can skate over the underside of skin and radiate through fascial planes. Pain can burn. It can make a person walk slowly or need a wheelchair. It can decide whether or not a person goes to school. It can determine whether or not one can bear children. Pain is a lived experience and it is a boundary that regulates existence. Learning to ask about what the pain feels like and what it means to the person experiencing it takes practice. A clinician who wants to treat HCTDs needs to learn how to speak the language of pain and to hear what is communicated.

Parsing out causes and expressions of pain can be tedious detail work, if we see it that way, or it can be an expression of the story of a person's life, if we opt to hear it another way. How we choose to listen and what we take from it will set the tone for subsequent interactions. My recommendation is that the clinician establishes that they want to understand and that they are a great listener but, equally, that they are careful not to dwell too long on this topic during the first appointment. It is a fine line and one that is easily crossed by the unwary, but we do not want to train our patients to trauma dump at appointments. If they are accustomed to doing so, then the appointment will no longer be a haven of respite from pain. Instead, it will become a place where the patient digs deep and experiences their suffering for a captive audience (the clinician). This, ultimately, helps no one.

We ask about the patient's current healthcare team. Some patients have been battered by Western medicine enough that they will make us their most trusted resource. Others live with extreme pain, require a team, and see Chinese medicine as a complementary modality. If their pain management exceeds my scope of practice, then I'm glad not to be centered. For those who do not want anything to do with biomedicine, I'm happy to be a resource.[15]

## Elimination (Urine and Stool)

Unless the patient suffers from gastroparesis or MCAS, bowel movement history is similar to that of any other patient. Some people struggle with constipation, others with diarrhea. Some folks want to lose weight. Others have diabetes or metabolic syndrome. An EDS patient with celiac disease or gluten intolerance will not differ radically from a patient who comes in for reasons other than connective tissue disorder.

The elimination norms of a person with MCAS often have an accompanying symptom or sign. Generally, the patient will have not only the constipation or diarrhea but also something other that indicates a systemic revolt against the offending item, be it a smell or food or chemical. In other words, we will want to ask about constipation (or diarrhea or whatever) *and what else?* This could be hives, it could be rolling waves of panic, it could be angioedema at the smell of food, it could be a person's soft palate peeling off if they eat anything hot. What else accompanies the bowel sign? The task for a practitioner is to determine where the bowel movement issue fits. In so doing, we identify differences between, say, a yang qi deficiency presentation (aka gastroparesis) vs. an issue pertaining to Wind (MCAS) or perhaps yin Fire (an aspect of the EDS syndrome related to Spleen qi and yang deficiency).

Urination patterns hold clues. When the bladder is weak or prolapsed, incomplete emptying can lead to chronic urinary tract infections (UTIs). Ptosis can be a factor. If the patient has to urinate multiple times during the night, it may be because the organs are shifting and pressure on the bladder makes them wake; combine this with MCAS and cell degranulation in the bladder, and a patient may need to urinate four, five, six, or more times during the night, indicating Cold and yang deficiency in combination with Spleen qi sinking.

Either way, asking about urination is important. Color and odor may not be of great importance in the EDS intake but frequency and whether or not it is painful will give us information that we need to know.

## Digestion (Thirst, Appetite, Tastes)

The relative strength or weakness of the digestive system in an EDS patient requires attention. The Spleen regulates the muscles of the body and the Liver is in control of the sinews. It is unsurprising to see a Liver overacting on Spleen presentation. A swollen or geographic tongue is not unusual. A taste for sweet rather than salty may be expected in the absence of POTS; otherwise, if there is any form of orthostatic intolerance, the patient will generally crave salt. We can acquire a good bit of wisdom by asking if the patient drinks pickle juice or craves the liquid from the jar more so than the olives if given a choice.

Nausea, lack of appetite, and weak digestion are fairly common in hEDS patients. This is unsurprising given the relation of the Spleen to the Stomach. Lack of sufficient nutrition then leads to Blood deficiency. Fatigue can be traced back to weakness of the digestive system. Nurturing digestion can be the sole focus of treatment and even doing just that can make a difference for a patient's wellbeing. We can expect to spend a good amount of time during the initial intake on questions and answers relating to digestive history.

## Sleep

A patient with a weak neck may suffer from sleep apnea; if the cervical spine is unstable, the patient may have issues because the throat is squeezed during sleep. Some patients will pop their ribs out by turning over in their sleep or they sublux a major joint.

Being unable to exercise may mean that the patient remains at a constant state of low-level anxiety that movement could remedy...if only they were able to get their heart pumping with regular movement. They are tired and wired or have brain fog... but they do not sleep well and, lacking refreshing sleep, a cycle is set in motion that is difficult to undo.

It is extremely hard to fall asleep when one is in pain. Even if one is exhausted enough to fall asleep, one does not stay asleep when pain is overwhelming. Months of this sort of interruption can wreak havoc on multiple systems of the body. A monkey mind that never rests is exhausting. It may be that the patient has, like so many people in this world, suffered trauma. Vivid dreams and night terrors are possible here.

Waking up in the middle of the night to urinate multiple times can make restorative sleep an impossible dream.

Our thorough understanding of sleep and how sleep disorder affects the patient is significant. Being able to sleep decently even occasionally can change things immeasurably. It is important during initial intake or soon thereafter to gain a meaningful understanding of the patient's sleep history and patterns.

## Thorax and Abdomen

Answers to questions regarding pain, bloating, and other discomfort can be useful in that they help to determine Liver qi stagnation, for instance, or Dampness in the lower Jiao. An hEDS patient can have the sighing and costal tightness that we associate with Liver qi stagnation, the chest tightness that we could attribute to Blood stasis of the Heart, or the bloated middle that we would identify as disorder of Spleen and Stomach. However, in a person with hEDS, this may be due to dysfunctional connective tissue rather than a sign of what we traditionally identify as a pattern attached to organ or organ function.

## Gynecological (and Men's Health Questions)

The ten questions refer to gynecological concerns and not to men's health. For people with hEDS, there are specific concerns that affect both male and female reproductive systems. Thus, I add men's health to this section.

For patients who have female reproductive systems, questions surrounding menstrual history and process do not have radically different answers from an EDS vs. a non-EDS patient, though endometriosis tends to strike hard in the former. What affects people with EDS, male reproductive systems or female, is prolapse. Most patients work with a pelvic floor specialist, and our ability to nurture Spleen qi can support their efforts. After surgery to repair the pelvic floor, we can nurture the healing process. A practitioner who specializes in women's health or fertility will certainly become familiar with prolapse.[16] Male patients experience erectile dysfunction. Rectal prolapse can be a problem for male and female EDS patients.

We need to be comfortable asking about tenesmus, erectile dysfunction, down-bearing pressure on the pelvic floor, and any other reproductive-system symptoms that seem relevant. It may be tethered cord, it may be Spleen qi sinking, or it could be many different things, but these are issues that are common in this patient population. And yes, most times the patient will be diagnosed by a gynecologist or urologist and be in treatment with a pelvic floor PT or a surgeon. But we can help our patients to live better, more comfortable lives by being aware of the challenges to pelvic floor and reproductive health posed by hEDS.

## History (Medical, Familial, Drug Use/ Supplements, Emotional States)

Completing a thorough medical history without going off on tangents requires tact and focus. As practitioners of Chinese medicine, we make time for our patients in a way that an MD may not be able to do, especially if they are bound by the strictures of insurance. However, if not planned well, the intake with an EDS patient can ricochet in five directions and go nowhere.

Family history is important. EDS is a heritable disorder, so often, though not always, there is someone in the family who has shown signs of it. Supplements and prescriptions require attention. Some patients cannot take anything without hyper-reactivity, and the phrase "low and slow" is popular in EDS circles because a practitioner really does have to start with half or quarter doses of everything. If it is not an issue of MCAS then it could be a matter of poor metabolism of drugs; either way, the patient's drug history speaks volumes. As I illuminate in subsequent chapters, a patient's mood may be related to their context or it could be a response to a dysregulated autonomic nervous system.

Learning to focus the intake and to pace what information to follow takes practice. It is all necessary information. The problem is that there really is a lot of it.

## III. Five Elements, Six Stages, Eight Principles: Which Door First?

Interpreting or categorizing the content of the ten (or thousand) questions a practitioner asks is not just a matter of *bian bing* vs. *bian zheng*. Of the multiple diagnostic models available to us, some are more relevant and useful than others when it comes to treating HCTD. Others become more useful when placing the common comorbidities such as MCAS and POTS. Before addressing specific approaches in the chapter subsequent to this one, I acknowledge pertinent diagnostic models and illuminate how they can be used to achieve a meaningful diagnosis. I also invite consideration of the Sixty-First Difficult Issue outlined in the *Nan-Ching*. Its opening declaration regarding the relative prowess of the physician states that, "Anybody who looks and knows it is to be called a spirit" (Unschuld 1986, p.539). What does this mean? Before addressing specific approaches in the next chapter, I share my thoughts on this complicated issue.

A diagnosis based on the Eight Principles is based on the relative engagement of four opposing pairs: yin and yang, Hot and Cold, internal and external, and excess or deficiency. What complicates this process when treating hEDS and comorbid conditions is that the hEDS norm is a challenge to establish. An Eight Principles approach is one that we will almost always use, but (as with *bian bing*) it becomes less reliable in terms of the larger picture of hEDS. What stabilizes an Eight Principles approach is the understanding of *what that patient's norm is*, all things considered. Not what a *standard* norm is but, rather, an *HCTD* norm. This is individual to each patient, but each patient has one.

A Six Evils (Wind, Cold, Heat, Dampness, Dryness, and Summer Heat) approach requires translation to the norms of the hEDS body on its own terms as well. For instance, MCAS is a matter of Wind but it is reflective of what I call wei qi rebellion.[17] The patient is deficient, if by deficient we mean that the pathogen is strong and the response is weak. However, in the case of MCAS, the pathogen can be weak but the wei qi ungovernable in response to one random stimulus. To other stimuli, it may be completely indifferent. Dampness and Phlegm patterns are similar to those in a non-hEDS patient but whether these are internally generated or an external threat becomes a more pressing question when piecing together a syndrome. The broad view of a Six Evils diagnosis starts our process, but its ultimate benefit rests on the practitioner's ability to assess the normative baseline of the hEDS body on an individual basis.

In my experience, more fruitful diagnostic models for an hEDS patient rely on the zangfu and channel diagnostics approaches, though the two basics that I have just mentioned are always part of the discernment process. Choosing a specific organ and deciding that it will be the one against which the others will be evaluated can be a viable option. But are we looking at an organ or the concept of an organ as an umbrella category? A straightforward view ("Liver overacting on Spleen," for instance) might work for one context but do nothing for the bigger picture. This is, after all, a matter of the pre-natal jing and how it constructed the resulting body. Where these pathways lead, via the channels, is unstable but, at the very least, will provide a tangible map that a practitioner might follow.[18]

As ever, we consider patient before disease. There are two very different patient types to keep in mind. One is the diagnosed patient. Someone might come in stating that they have been diagnosed with hEDS, POTS, MCAS, and gastroparesis. This patient wants to try acupuncture for pain relief and digestive support. The practitioner, already knowing what the patient "has," can readily begin with a *bian bing* focus. That seems straightforward. It is not. What if the patient "has" MALS and their doctor hasn't caught it? Tracking symptoms and applying a *bian zheng* approach, one that closely monitors channels and organ, can help a practitioner to decipher shifts in that patient's presentation. In so doing, we spot red flags and are able to urge follow-up with the appropriate MD in such cases. If syndrome pattern contradicts disease identification, this is an invitation to reconsider and decide whether or not there are safety issues at hand.

What about the patient who is undiagnosed? Someone comes in because they have neck pain or a twisted ankle that has been deemed not broken by the orthopedic surgeon. Perhaps a diagnosis of Bi syndrome is appropriate. But, upon palpation, the practitioner realizes that the patient is hypermobile. A string of signs and symptoms all pan out and, sure enough, it becomes clear that the patient could benefit from a diagnosis of hEDS or JHS. Depending then on what the patient wants, perhaps they will go back to their MD. It might also be possible that the patient is not interested in a biomedical diagnosis and does not need one in order for the practitioner to remain within scope of practice. Running through a *bian bing* checklist of sorts, the practitioner can decide what is safe to treat and proceed from there by setting aside disease category in favor of a focus on imbalance. With this scenario, the practitioner is going to look closer at syndromes and patterns, and knowingly focus less on a specific disease diagnosis.

As long as the patient is diagnosed or not showing red flags, it is perfectly possible to bypass the label of hEDS entirely and simply focus on the syndrome. In so doing, we offer the patient options and differing strategies for treating their conditions. The way an MCAS or hEDS patient can hyper-react to pharmaceutical drugs (or not react as expected) means that we prescribe herbal formulas and often do quite well for them. Deconstructing the interrelations of the body's systems may not give us the answer that a genetic identifier would, but we are still able to discern in an excellent fashion. We have valuable strategies. There is no one right answer unless the patient is showing red flags for conditions that are out of one's scope of practice.

And so, we arrive at the Sixty-First Difficult Issue. Herein, "The scripture states: Anybody who looks and knows it is to be called a spirit; anybody who listens and knows it is to be called a sage; anybody who asks and knows it is to be called an artisan; anybody who feels the vessels and knows it is to be called a skilled workman. What does that mean?" (*ibid.*, p.539). The commentary that follows includes remarks such as, "A spirit looks at the [patient] and knows [his illness]; he does not have to ask him..." (p.539) and, "One knows the illness before it becomes manifest" (p.543). It reveals the worth of the practitioner. Yet do we need to ask questions and palpate, or can one just know? I read this while in my program and reviewed it while writing this book. As I develop as a practitioner, I see how it begins to take less to know more. Knowing the right questions to ask is to be a sage, to be sure. But what of looking and simply knowing? What is it that we must know?[19]

When treating patients, part of the knowing is being capable of seeing a human being. Where is the individual in terms of their own feeling about their diagnosis (or lack), their degree of disability, or their sense of self as a person with a complex disorder? What does the patient need, and what might help them to be more at ease in their larger context? Maybe the person does not know the answers to these questions, but when we are receptive listeners, our chances of supporting the patient as they figure them out is greater. How many times have any one of us tried to communicate a heartfelt message but experienced the pain of not being understood? When we feel invisible, we feel a deep sense of hurt. How can anyone heal if they are not truly seen?

Especially after the first years of the COVID pandemic, so many of us have experienced loneliness and isolation. In some countries (my own, for example), people in medically vulnerable communities are feeling injured and overlooked by the notion that masks are no longer necessary (at least according to those who want to happily declare that, "COVID is over—it's nothing more than a flu!"). The venerated medical ancestor, Li Dong-Yuan, saw that his patient population was a traumatized one. Ours is today. Will we actually see them? A practitioner who can truly see a patient and who can genuinely hear that person when they communicate is a spirit. To ask and to sincerely, genuinely listen is the work of not just a sage but also a saint. Practitioners of Chinese medicine may have more time for their initial intake than an MD and we can take pride in the length of our appointments. It is true that we can be a safe harbor for patients who have been so badly treated that they suffer from medical PTSD. But we are not perfect either. We all can practice and cultivate our spirit and sage-like qualities.

Though the difficult question pertains to seeing colors of the face and making a correct diagnosis, it is worth viewing through the lens of how profoundly our patients need to be seen. It is worth viewing through the lens of self-mastery, too. Our patients with hEDS need that extra refinement from us. And really, is it not so that all patients (and we, too, are patients) need excellence from those who take on the duty of our care? The tale of Bian Qu who saw the marquis Qi Huan's illness before it manifested is held as an example of this legendary physician's gift for preventative treatment. We may not be able to prevent or cure a hereditary illness but we certainly can, simply by listening and by truly seeing, nourish the souls of our patients. This is a valuable skill.[20]

Do we need to see a disease category? Should we, rather, look for patterns? I think we first can look at the person, one who lives with a complex disorder. What does this person need? What might we give to them? I believe that we need to go back and forth between identifying a disease and practicing critical thought via the identification of syndromes and patterns. I also think that we need to genuinely listen to our patients and to look at them with eyes that see the needs of a human being who lives with an HCTD. In my estimation, we must ask ourselves daily, and before each patient, how is it that we will choose to see?

Difficult questions, indeed.

How we arrive at a diagnosis depends on many factors. Once we have made our choices and identified the pattern or categorized the disease, it is then most efficacious to pick a realm and mindfully start from there. Consequently, in the next chapter, I address four routes of treatment. These are: Bi syndrome, via the precepts of the Earth School, with a focus on the shen, or through the lens of Gu syndrome.

# CHAPTER 3

# A Hypermobile Heroic Journey

## I. Map-Making, with Miles to Go

People who live with chronic illness often become their own best advocates. Online communities, especially, are rewriting cultural narratives about what it means to live with chronic illness and/or pain. The main part of this chapter outlines four approaches that constitute logical potential starting points; beginning with one or more can give practitioners freedom to move within a diagnostic framework. But surrounding this practical consideration are significant questions. How do we communicate with our patients, and how do we become better listeners? How might we consider what HCTDs mean to those who live with them, and in what ways would this matter as we build practices that welcome people with chronic disorders? A digression into the anthropology of disability is beyond the scope of this discussion, but the topic is relevant and we enlarge our perspective when we acknowledge social groups and cultural shifts.[1]

Where do we go when we take part in their journey? Unique presentations that shift, alter, and undergo metamorphosis at any and all new turns create obstacles when planning treatment. Context provides what a designated genotype cannot, and patients are embedded, intersectional beings (as are healthcare providers). Where the patient is in terms of what they know about their condition and how they experience the health concerns that bring them to the clinical encounter invites consideration. Without placing the patient and locating ourselves, we run the risk of chasing one symptom or sign after the next and not getting anywhere. Because these are people with multi-system dysfunctions, it can be difficult to find a place to begin.

We need to find that one thread and follow it. By choosing a home base, be it Bi syndrome, the Earth School, the shen, or Gu syndrome, and then by sticking with it, we avoid piecemeal or patchwork treatments. By placing the patient and their context into meaningful constructs, a practitioner is better positioned to map out a plan. Whether it is one of the four starting points I discuss in this chapter or something other, my hope is to offer a useable blueprint. Finally, a practitioner also needs to further contextualize the patient when opting to prescribe herbal formulas (or not), as I discuss in the concluding section of this chapter.

Before considering any one of these options, we might pause for a moment and consider what brings hypermobile people to our clinics. What do they know about HCTDs or hEDS? How do they experience their bodies? What do they expect from Chinese medicine? Are they diagnosed? Any of the four options can work for an hEDS patient, but comprehension of the patient's subject position helps us to select the most appropriate one.

As we know, it is difficult to get a diagnosis of hEDS. An hEDS patient's diagnosis is a clinical one and it is stringent. Someone who is diagnosed with hEDS generally will have gotten so far because they are relatively disabled. Such a patient may have a wide array of medical care providers. They may have sought out Chinese medicine with the expectation that "getting acupuncture" is helpful for pain, insomnia, or some specific aspect of their presentation that does not respond well to the team they have in place. This type of patient can be easier or harder to work with, relative to the other types, depending on what kind of support they require and how they view Chinese medicine.

Horizons do narrow when a patient has been given a biomedical diagnosis and is comfortable within the biomedical system. This is not a bad thing. If the patient and the practitioner agree that the patient is there for pain, then the practitioner can identify a Bi syndrome and treat it. Having a PCP, a rheumatologist, a cardiologist, a urogynecologist, an orthopedic surgeon, a PT, a psychiatrist, a psychotherapist, and a nutritionist on board relieves us from feeling overwhelmed by a sense of responsibility for issues that may not even be in our scope of practice. What we do here is still valuable. Above and beyond treating for Bi syndrome, we also keep our eyes open for red flags and alert the patient so that they can go back to their biomedical team with concerns if needed. We can provide a safe, comfortable place to have a restful treatment. A diagnosed patient with a team of healthcare providers can be easy to work with because the boundaries are clear.

That said, it also depends. The first time a patient's PT performs the so-called dry needling on the patient and they come in with a ghastly bruise on a limb that the practitioner has successfully treated with acupuncture is jarring. My policy with patients who also see PTs is that they need to tell me if they opt to try this or trigger-point needling with the other practitioner. That way, I avoid working on the same region and I may decide to not treat the patient with acupuncture at all. I do not want to over treat an area and I'm disinclined to risk being unfairly blamed for bruises or untoward outcomes. I do not take this personally. If the patient is most comfortable being treated by biomedical practitioners, that is their right. What matters is that the Chinese medicine practitioner decides whether or not they want to be part of a program that includes dry or trigger-point needling by a PT. If they do not, then they need to be forthright about it.

Of the diagnosed, there will be a subset that consists of the self-diagnosed. These patients can be a joy to work with if the practitioner enjoys engaging with people who do their own research. I am still very much Professor Bruno, so a patient who does their own homework is a gem in my (grade)book. Not every practitioner is comfortable with this level of self-actualization. If we are, we need to be mindful about scope of practice. My experience has been that self-diagnosed patients who want to be as independent of biomedicine as possible are a joy to work with as long as they agree to acquiesce to referrals in the event of red flags or needs beyond what I am legally able to do. Such patients may have a functional medicine doctor to take responsibility for their primary care. As long as that MD sincerely respects Chinese medicine and does not try to concurrently supplant what we do via so-called "medical acupuncture," this can be an ideal scenario.[2]

These patients often want to address anxiety, gut health, or pain. In Texas, a licensed acupuncturist can treat certain issues without the patient having been seen by a dentist, chiropractor, or MD for that condition at least once within the previous year.[3] Chronic pain is one, and we are able to work meaningfully with these patients without the input of biomedicine if the focus is pain relief. Some self-diagnosed patients, in contrast to the above-described, come to the clinical encounter because they have been gaslit and abused by the biomedical system. These patients need support and encouragement. They need to be retaught lessons about efficacy and boundaries. Not all practitioners enjoy the role of teacher, but we who do will love guiding these marvelous, worthy patients as they begin to learn how to navigate their own health needs.

Undiagnosed patients bring their joys and challenges to the clinic. A patient with a mystery disease could very well have hEDS and MCAS. Some of these patients have been to an endless stream of specialists, to no avail. Is this a Gu presentation?

Maybe we should start with Bi syndrome. Whatever we do, we want to remain steady and not allow ourselves to go off on tangents. Trying to resolve everything or be the medical detective who figures out the case and saves the day might result in great success or it could end up with tears all around, if not worse.

I laughed when I read the translation of the *Complete Compendium of Zhang Jingyue, Vol. 1-3: Eight Principles, Ten Questions, and Mingmen Theory*. In the section "Although It Is Not a Difficult Affair to Diagnose and Make Judgment, One Must Also Be Wise, So as to Prevent the Incurrences of Enmity" (Zhang 2020, pp.153–156), Dr. Zhang, an apparently very opinionated Ming-dynasty physician, had wisdom to share regarding patients who go from one practitioner to the next. In his own words:

> There are those who mix up various types of modalities without any focus. They [listen to] Mr. Wáng in the morning and [listen to] Mr. Lǐ in the evening, without any judgement of their own. When they feel nothing with the prescribed medicinals, if they are subsequently misled by others, then they will readily abandon [the current physician] and yearn for another. For the next [physicians] in line, in order to display their superiority, they would comment on the shortcomings of the previous [physicians]. And when they fail, they would instead blame it on [the previous physicians]. (*ibid.*, p.154)

I have a lot of compassion for people who are medical mysteries, so my laughter was rueful and aware of why patients might behave this way. I am not as snappy and cranky as Dr. Zhang. But mystery patients in his time (1563–1640 CE) are a cautionary tale for those of us who practice today. His commentary offers a reminder of the wisdom of choosing an approach and sticking with a plan. In chapter six, I reference excellent illness memoirs that bring to life the genuine suffering that medical-mystery patients experience and make it clear why they had little choice but to go from one practitioner to another. For now, it suffices to make two declarations. First: there is much that a compassionate practitioner can do for medical-mystery patients; second: to pick a thread and follow it is the smartest and safest tactic, both for patient and for practitioner.

Undiagnosed and oblivious patients can be heartbreaking.

When a patient comes in for insomnia or low back pain, these are conditions that do not carry extra baggage. Granted, common ailments can make a person's life miserable if they are severe. But these are known entities. When it comes to HCTD, what can I say other than *here be dragons*? It is hard to tell someone who came in for treatment of low back pain to ask their MD about Marfan syndrome. Marfan syndrome carries with it an increased risk for cardiac disease. If diagnosed, they need to manage their health under the supervision of a specialist. It is hard to tell someone that their erectile dysfunction that did not respond to testosterone therapy may possibly be part of an hEDS presentation and that they might want to take a list of their signs and symptoms to their MD. They come in with an embarrassing condition only to find out that it might be associated with a life-long chronic disorder.

An oblivious patient may need to be pointed towards diagnosis, or they could have enough information if they simply understand their own bodies. Either way, safety requires a practitioner who is observant and knowledgeable. A patient with no red flags can be eased into knowledge of hypermobility. Without giving too much information at once and by parceling it out in manageable amounts, we can teach the patient self-awareness so that they eventually feel like they have figured their situation out for themselves. Then they can proceed accordingly and maintain a sense of control over their process of self-discovery. A patient with red flags needs direct intervention and different forms of support. They may need help to plan what to say to their MD and they may need guidance as they put puzzle pieces together and ultimately learn what it is that has been causing so many health concerns for so long.

When a practitioner has a clear idea of where the patient is, in terms of what they know and what they need, this is one of the most genuine forms of seeing—as per the previous chapter—that we can cultivate. We are spirits when we see our patients as they need to be seen.

And with this clear vision, the practitioner is ready to begin planning a healthcare strategy that is safe, effective, and reflective of the very best that Chinese medicine has to offer. Once again, it is a matter of choosing a thread and following it. As Dr. Liu reminds, "All roads lead to Beijing" (2019, p.385).[4]

## II. Wide Open Fields and Mindful Approaches: Bi, the Earth School, Shen, and Gu

### Bi Syndrome

Pain that lasts for three months or more is a line item on the list of diagnostic criteria for EDS patients. With or without diagnosis, a person with hypermobile joints and a range of comorbid conditions is intimately acquainted with pain. The decision to identify Bi syndrome as the primary point of departure is entirely non-controversial, and a practitioner who does so is able to justify it on many grounds.

What Bi syndrome means for an HCTD patient requires an adjusted lens. A body with EDS has its version of normal, and knowing what that is creates possibilities for meaningful treatment. When we study anatomy and physiology, we begin in an excellent position to be of service to the HCTD communities. However, it is more important to know the anatomy of muscle, bone, tendon, and ligament as they normally are *for someone with EDS*. We must develop our understanding of fascia and the lymphatic system in this manner too. With a firm grasp of the normative EDS physical body as it is framed by its own narrative and expressed via its faulty gene, we are then able to return to Chinese medicine's construction of meaning and matter. We are, in so doing, able to provide treatment that is safe and effective and reflective of Chinese medicine's value system and strengths.

What is pain to someone with hEDS or extremely mobile joints? When we speak of Bi, we move into the realm of rheumatology. We also enter into an experience that is objective on the pragmatic end and subjective from the side of lived experience.

It's common for people with EDS to have a high pain tolerance; in its absence, one could not survive. A person who reacts normally to an abnormally high level of pain would not be able to function. Social factors, perhaps medical gaslighting, fear of being fired by an impatient boss, or maybe compassion fatigue causing loved ones to be unsupportive, all contribute to a sufferer's decision to learn to quietly live with pain. Shame may be a consideration. It can be humiliating to suffer so; a person may view chronic pain as a weakness to be hidden. Maybe it is frightening to be in pain, so the person has learned to pretend that it does not exist. Finally, if pain is all one knows, it becomes hard to judge when the pain has crossed a boundary into dangerous territories. Pain is, therefore, something that we (and we will all know pain one day), the ones who endure it, might not even have words to express.

A practitioner who can see this is a spirit indeed.

A practitioner who works with hEDS can apply the same considerations for pain treatment to hEDS patients that would be extended to pain patients in general. Hot or Cold? Wandering or fixed? Is this Blood stasis or is it Phlegm and Dampness based? None of the principles of etiology are radically different between a pain patient and a pain patient with hEDS. There are differences though, and these are due to particular characteristics of hEDS. For pain that afflicts the entire body, it can be extraordinarily challenging to determine root cause, especially if the branches are thorny and overly intertwined. A practitioner needs to learn how to decipher a patient's own language of pain in order to address it meaningfully. Teaching the patient to identify and gauge pain levels is an important task. The pain of hEDS is a hydra of its own. We have fairly clear (at least to us) languages for determining causes of Bi syndrome; patients, for their part, often struggle to speak and be heard when navigating the expression of what it means, to that individual, to be in pain.

Consider, for example, the difference between subluxation and dislocation. The latter is when two bones of a joint are separated to the extent that they no longer touch each other; the former is, for its part, a relatively minor form of dislocation wherein the joint surfaces touch but are not in their correct alignment with one another. When a person's joints separate and bone slides from bone, this can be excruciating or it can be annoying. For some, this is a daily occurrence. For others, it is occasional. For some, it is extremely disabling. For others, it is painful but, with effort, can be ignored. No medical intervention or tradition—not Eastern, not Western—can turn joints like these into so-called normal, properly functioning ones. But by understanding that particular patient's "normal," a practitioner can enhance what is possible to improve and nurture what is working well with the aim of building on the patient's strengths. A well-considered Bi syndrome approach is a worthy one if it is constructed via the norms of EDS.

My personal experience with a particular joint is instructive. Leaving aside my knee that has subluxed more times than I can count (it's not that interesting a story), I will say that I am the only person I know personally who subluxed a femur just by stretching. This occurred when I was in my first graduate program. I worked in the student gym in the weight room and did my own workouts there as well. One day, after an excellent session, I went to the stretching area and put my leg up on a ledge and easily put my nose to my kneecap. I was warmed up, feeling really good, and I didn't take care the way I normally would. The stretch felt so marvelous that I relaxed right into it...until I heard a sound like a chicken leg being popped off the carcass and felt a tearing sensation as the structures holding my femur in place broke apart. I stood, shocked, a wave of sudden sweat pouring out of my body, and then I shifted slightly so that my leg fell off the ledge. As it did so, my joint snapped back in the socket and the tissue surrounding it swelled up so that I felt like I had a breast implant under my butt cheek medial to my hamstrings.

Like anyone accustomed to this sort of weirdness, I did the normal thing that life had taught me to do: I decided that I was fine and gingerly tiptoed out of the gym. Halfway down the walkway and just before the information desk where my coworkers hung out, I sat at one of the machines because the pain was so incredible that I was forced to stop and catch my breath before walking by anyone I knew. I managed to hide the fact that I was in agony and I made it home by sheer force of will. Driving a stick shift, as I do, is not easy under such circumstances, but I managed. I would pay for this, of course. For months, my femur was unstable. When it finally healed, I suffered pain, sometimes mild and other times severe, with every step for the following nearly twenty years until I started getting treatment from my teacher, Dr. Fan.

I didn't know any better than to do what I did. This is what I was used to and it was not a tremendous shock to feel my bones separate. Sure, it was astonishing to have it be a femur, and yes, the swelling and the bruising indicated that something had torn (actually, the tearing noise and excruciating pain also were messages) but my knee had popped out several times in my life and I never questioned that this was normal. It was normal for me, anyway.

One of my first very long-term patients, on the other hand, came to me via referral from her doctor. This patient had a loose hip joint and suffered chronic pain. She had been sent to a PT initially but was not happy about it. She thought that the PT was rough and uncaring and was afraid that I would hurt her too. Her tongue was pale and her pulse thin and weak. She had a Lyme-disease history and was always, always afraid that each and every pain meant the end of the line for her. Her hip joint did feel like it could be popped out without much effort. Her constitution was fragile and her constant fear of illness bore fruit. She experienced one strange episode of poor health after the next and it would have been very easy, especially since I was but a junior practitioner at the time, to go off on tangents. I managed to refrain only because I knew that it was best for her that we had a singular goal in mind.

I saw her twice a week for a year and our focus was her pain. A Bi syndrome diagnosis kept us on track and she was able to improve immeasurably just by coming in and concentrating on one thing: pain resolution. I supported qi, warmed channels, and boosted yang. I nourished her Kidneys (one of which was floating, as confirmed by an MD) and added ear seeds to shen-men to help her to feel calmer. This was, in my estimation, an undiagnosed hEDS case, and no, I could not cure that. But when my patient eventually began to experience less discomfort and more efficacy within her own body, the overwhelming fear dissipated. Yes, she still had loose joints and was often in pain, but she was less fearful and more able to live within the body that was hers. In my estimation, this was a successful outcome and she felt the same way too.

Subluxation can also be like my patients with joints that seem simply to disintegrate. The tissue feels like cornsilk and on palpation, it is easy to feel that the tissue is soft and weak. Others, like my patient with the loose hip joint, feel like their tendons are slippery rubber bands. Someone who has torn out a femur or popped out a knee might not have that cornsilk feel to their tendons (I don't) but what they have, instead, is a lifetime of being slightly off-center due to compensating for the original injury. They may have internal scarring around the joint that is locally painful and which results in dysfunction along the relevant kinetic chain. Some patients will come in already knowing that it is not normal to pop out their joints, and others will need to be educated. Everyone is different.

The in-between that many hEDS people know is neither the cornsilk tendons that give way at will nor the tear of a major joint and the scarring that follows. Instead, it is the challenge of perennially loose joints that allow for slippage and grinding in the interstices. It could be fingers that require splints. It's the spine, maybe, that curves, or spondylosis. A person with HCTD will have the same health concerns that any other person would have as they age, too. Bad posture, text neck, sports injuries that don't heal properly? People with hEDS have those too, just worse, usually. Trigger fingers, thumbs, and even trigger toes are not surprising in hEDS patients. It is not unusual to see cases where the patient's ankle (usually one, not both) spasms and then twists, hard. This can be excruciating. My patients with trigger finger usually have more than one affected digit.

The pain of weak, cold, flaccid body parts (Cold Bi) is common in hEDS patients, especially in the distal joints, the fingers and toes, or in the lower back. Another relatively common scenario relates to fibromyalgia. Patients diagnosed with fibromyalgia are often undiagnosed cases of hEDS and this can result in psychological pain that exacerbates the physical. If a practitioner works with fibromyalgia, it can be useful to pay attention to the patient's joints and their flexibility. Fibromyalgia sometimes is simply fibromyalgia. When it is actually hEDS, a practitioner will do their patients a service by helping them get diagnosed (if that is what they want) or, at the very least, supporting them in becoming more informed and thus able to expand their horizons, treatment wise.

To be able to genuinely see the space between what pain

"sounds like" to the clinician vs. what it is "lived like" via the patient requires our curiosity and respect. We need to listen to the patient's story and we need to hear it in their language, not ours. The patient knows what happens but may not know that what they experience is not "normal." A practitioner who treats from the starting point of Bi syndrome also needs to learn the tangible and unspoken expressive language of an hEDS body. If not, it can be dangerous. We imagine what might happen if we perform a range of motion (ROM) test on a patient. That could result in a shocking injury. But when there is excellent communication? This is when substantive progress can be made.

We cannot "cure" these patients. What we can do, instead, is learn to meaningfully navigate their version of normal. Avoiding ROM tests in favor of gentle palpation is helpful. We pay attention to the way they express pain and learn to hear their language of it. Becoming very aware of the issues that are uncommon to the general population but extremely common to people with hEDS is crucial. The very nature of HCTDs places them within the category of Bi syndromes, and Chinese medicine is especially valuable to treat intractable pain. As long as the practitioner understands hEDS and adjusts their lens to accommodate it, an approach that begins via the purview of Bi syndrome can be ideal.

## Centering the Earth

Some days, my patient roster trends towards a theme.

The first patient of the day has tendons like cornsilk and fascia like water. When she reaches—to open a door, to grab something off a shelf, to hug a loved one—without thinking, her shoulder disintegrates. She has a bloated abdomen and complains of nausea, reflux, belching, and gas. She is constipated.

The second patient has stretchy skin and cigarette-paper scars. No history of subluxation but she is remarkably flexible and has experienced a lifetime of chronic pain, especially in her neck from the juncture of skull and spine all the way to the C-7 vertebra. She has hemorrhoids and tends to have three bowel movements daily. Like the first patient, she is on the thin side.

The third patient has the same silky exterior as the second. She's got a little more padding on her bones—though she is in no way overweight—and no history of subluxations or formal diagnosis, but her medical history is littered with clues. She had surgery for a lipoma that left her scarred and in worse condition than before the intervention. Though her abs are flat, she is constipated. When she does have a bowel movement, which happens maybe every ten days, the issue is paltry. Where does her digested food go? Multiple GI doctors and varying scans and scopes and tests have not provided any answers. She too suffers from hemorrhoids.

Later, a soft-skinned former gymnast will come in for their weekly treatment. They are here for constipation and pain relief (they have a shoulder that is loose and no amount of physical therapy or orthopedic intervention has helped). They are chronically anxious. They have one bowel movement a week, if that. Just before their period, they have a veritable deluge that leaves them feeling as though their insides will come out along with the suddenly unclogged waste.

All of these patients have pale, puffy tongues with a shiny clear coating and scalloped edges. Their pulses run soft and slightly faster than one might expect under the circumstances.

Over the course of the week, I see patients who cannot eat anything but a limited range of foods. Some get hives if they stray from the approved foods list, or their noses run, or they wheeze. Others bloat up and feel their intestines burning as their bodies attempt to digest anything but a tiny amount of food in one sitting. Others become incredibly anxious and experience debilitating psycho-emotional reactions to things like chocolate or dairy.

Leaving aside discussion of the Spleen and Stomach channels and acupuncture points for the chapter after this one, it suffices here to focus specifically on these organs in their relation to syndrome, pattern, and the larger picture of hypermobile healthcare. Whether we speak of the gut microbiome and chronic inflammation or we couch our discourse in the language of Phlegm, Dampness, and Spleen qi, we address systemic debility by starting in the middle Jiao. When working with hEDS, a practitioner will by default become an expert of the Earth School of Chinese medicine.

I am referring, of course, to venerable medical ancestor Li Dong-Yuan and his theories regarding the Spleen. As we recollect, Li Dong-Yuan (1180–1251) was the scion of a wealthy family. Known also as Li Gao, his upbringing and cultural context deeply influenced his development as a practitioner. He lived during a time of social upheaval and Mongol conquest and ultimately came to view an injured digestive system as the source of many, if not most, diseases. When we consider CTDs and HCTDs, it is always worth our time to refresh our memories about this important figure in Chinese medical history. His theories that became what we know as the Earth School are the result of his context. A practitioner today is able to extrapolate from his history in a useful manner (and not just for hEDS patients).

Li Dong-Yuan held that damage to Spleen and Stomach could be internally generated. The damaged Spleen and Stomach are unable to complete their tasks of intaking food and drink and transforming the food into qi. He further postulated that unresolved emotions related to poor digestive function leads to a cycle of rumination and internal disorder. Ultimately, what Li Dong-Yuan theorized in his day is what we see today in clinic as chronic inflammation and, at its most extreme, MCAS.

If we start from the perspective of the Earth School, we note that dysfunction is not always a matter of intemperate eating and drinking. Especially in the instance of MCAS, these are often people who can't eat much of anything. What they do have that sets them within Li Dong-Yuan's theories is exhaustion that manifests its discontent via the digestive processes. These are people who probably have congenitally weak Spleen qi to begin with; in addition, the taxation of living within a body that is constitutionally less than robust is wearying. In effect, HCTDs can entail a constant and chronic level of stress that is internalized until it causes yin Fire and other ill effects. In addition, near-nonexistent yang qi in the middle Jiao can lead to delayed gastric emptying. Whether it is called "gastroparesis" or "yang qi deficiency," it is common for someone with hEDS to have slow digestion.

If a practitioner chooses to approach the treatment of hEDS via the middle Jiao, it is crucial to keep the more significant red flags in mind. Compression disorders such as the ones I outline in chapter one (e.g., MALS and nutcracker syndrome) are rare, they are hard to diagnose, and it may be challenging for patients to find doctors who know about them. A Chinese medicine practitioner who works with HCTDs, consequently, needs to be mindful when it comes to GI problems that may seem commonplace (nausea, lack of appetite, mild pain after eating) but which do not respond well to herbal and acupuncture treatment. People with HCTDs experience compression disorders. It is our responsibility to learn about the signs and symptoms and refer to an MD accordingly.

We will also remain cognizant of the effect of pharmaceutical interventions. Patients with ostensible chronic UTIs might be, instead, dealing with ptosis and inflammation. Someone with traveler's diarrhea or gastroenteritis might evince volatile symptoms as a result of their connective tissue's relative lack of strength. In either instance, their doctor might choose an antibiotic that is dangerous for them. A new patient came to my office, for example, and his chief complaint was wrist pain. Upon palpation, I noticed that his joints were loose and that the ligaments felt thin. As we went through his health history, I was alarmed to hear that he had just returned from Latin America with stomach pain that his primary care physician opted to treat with ciprofloxacin. He had not yet started taking his pills but had already picked them up at a pharmacy. I asked if his PCP had tried anything else first and the patient said no, that the PCP thought he had a parasite or giardia and that the cipro should fix it quickly.

It took all I had to sustain a peaceful mien as I asked if the pharmacist had discussed potential side effects with him. The patient said no, nobody had mentioned side effects.

I do not ever get between a patient and their doctor's prescriptions. Never. Doing so leaves me responsible for the patient's choice, and if the patient goes off a prescribed medication and the outcome is dire, I am then potentially liable. The only thing I will do when I disagree with a medication is suggest that the patient review potential side effects and discuss their concerns with a pharmacist or with their doctor. This patient caught my expression of horror and decided to (a) follow up with a pharmacist immediately after leaving their appointment with me and (b) upon doing so, he opted not to start taking the cipro. At our next appointment, he thanked me for not trying to argue him out of taking the drug but laughed when he mentioned the look on my face when he said the word "ciprofloxacin."

Hyperflexible people should avoid the class of antibiotics known as fluoroquinolones, of which cipro is one. As of 2018 in the United States, the Centers for Disease Control and Prevention (CDC) has added a black box warning about this class of antibiotics and their risks to people with connective tissue disorder. When a Chinese medicine practitioner starts working with HCTD patients, it is prudent to not become involved in what their MD prescribes. However, if it is a fluoroquinolone, the practitioner is within their scope of practice to educate about the dangers that such drugs pose. That this class of antibiotics is potentially dangerous to hypermobile people is not up for argument. It is a fact. Other medications that an MD might prescribe for GI disorders are considerably less dangerous than cipro but we still have options to offer hEDS patients, especially if we work from the perspective of Li Dong-Yuan. By making the Spleen and Stomach our focus, we not only can support digestion. We also might save a patient from potential harm.[5]

We might also be called upon to strengthen the middle Jiao so that the patient can better metabolize nutrients. Patients with extraordinarily weak digestion and hEDS may need to be fitted with an enteral feeding tube (also known as a J port). Most times, such patients will have a nutritionist who has been assigned to them via their gastroenterologist's office. However, Western biomedicine's nutritionists hold different theories than ours regarding food and its healing properties.[6] We may have patients who welcome education regarding Chinese medical nutrition if they are trying to avoid being fitted with a J port. An Earth nurturing approach can be useful here but, as with any significant disorder, success requires patience, consistency, and time to effect change.[7]

Some patients will be fat or obese. A person with chronic pain and unstable joints may not be able to exercise. Some people do; others cannot. Obesity rates are rising the world over due to a variety of causes, and it is erroneous to correlate HCTD with weight. Fatness in hEDS patients is due to all the normal reasons that are bringing up obesity rates worldwide. And yet, it may also be true that fatness in chronic illness patients is because the ostensible cause (inactivity, poor nutrition, overeating) is compounded by stress, pain, and possibly chronic inflammation.

Before addressing the matter of weight, there are contextual topics to consider. One is that the patient may have been told that their pain is all due to their weight and that they wouldn't suffer from joint pain if they lost a few pounds (or kilos or stones). Just like anyone else, a larger hEDS patient may have been belittled by other healthcare providers. The patient doesn't need it from their Chinese medicine practitioner, too. If the patient is large and has joint pain and difficulty getting around, how do we (or do we) discuss this with them? What is our honest philosophy of weight and size? Do we feel able to speak about HAES (health at every size)? If we can do so sincerely, then we are in a fine position to speak about weight and health with a patient. If not, it is probably a good idea to not begin from the starting point of nurturing Earth.[8]

If a practitioner does feel that they can support fat patients with respect and complete acceptance, and if the patient does want to work with the practitioner on size and weight, then there are questions to raise with that patient. What is the purpose of their act of eating? Do they eat for calories, for nutrition, for self-comfort? Are they willing to try Chinese medicine's approach? If they are, do they need to move slowly when introducing new foods or can they jump right in and try a variety of things? We keep in mind that heavier patients may have been treated poorly and may be at risk of developing orthorexia or other forms of disordered eating.[9]

When our healing strategy follows the precepts of the Earth School, we are providing our patients with time-tested care. What matters in a Spleen/Stomach approach is that we remain aware of red flags, both biomedical and psycho-emotional. In so doing, we are able to provide meaningful care for patients that effects worthwhile change.

## Emotional Landscapes (the Shen)

A trite question, maybe, but a worthy one in this context: which came first, the chicken or the egg? As with most queries in Chinese medicine, the answer is: it depends.

Which comes first? Pain? Or the reaction to it? Again: it depends.

Most important? A clinician is not able to resolve the matter of EDS in and of itself, but we certainly are able to create a space within it that allows for ease of emotional turmoil and, in so doing, we nurture health and wellbeing. Again: when working with hEDS patients there are, as ever, specific considerations to keep in mind.

When a patient comes in with a tangible concern or a health condition that is at least relatively objective, the clinician generally does not need to delve into the gap between, as we say in semiotics, signifier and signified. The signifier, in the case of complex diseases, consists of the syndrome or pattern names. Liver qi stagnation or anger, Lung qi deficiency or grief, a Heart that, overheated, has overshot the mark on joy and launched on towards mania, ruminating and worry or Spleen qi damage, and/ or the last but not least notion of shock affecting Kidney qi are one thing. The signified, or the thing, is one thing to the patient and another to the practitioner. What happens when the patient presents with these conditions and how one frames the issue at hand can never entirely account for the space between what the terms indicate and what they mean to the person who lives with the conditions in question. That space in between constitutes an entirely different universe that is as large or as small as one wishes it to be; what matters most is that the practitioner is aware of it, and of self.

A practitioner who focuses on the psyche, or at least provides service to the wellbeing of a patient's mind-body-spirit axis will forgive me for appearing to speak in riddles. Working with complex chronic illness requires a certain level of flexibility and cultivation of the inner self on the part of the practitioner. How is the practitioner's own shen doing? Emotional boundaries protect both patient and practitioner. A patient's sense of safety and their consequent ability to heal in response to the clinician's efforts depend on the cultivation of a safe and bounded space. For this reason, addressing the question of why a practitioner would consider taking a psycho-emotional strategy as their starting point of necessity begins by focusing on context and on the practitioner.

Just as in the realm of national trauma, my scholarly specialty in my previous career, there are big-picture aspects of EDS that factor into the individual's lived experience. When we work with complex chronic illness, we may be called upon to bear witness to grief, fear, shame, and pain. Psychotherapists, like any other medical professional, have their areas of expertise. Working with chronic pain or illness patients is a specialty area for therapists the way eating disorders, say, or marital counseling are specialty areas. Unless the Chinese medicine practitioner is also a licensed therapist with extra training to work with chronic pain or illness, it is smarter and safer to know where the edges of one's scope of practice end and to remain, mindfully, within said boundaries. Best of all: we keep a referral list of psychotherapists and have an idea of where to refer if we feel that the patient needs help making meaning of their suffering.[10]

When we do address the psyche in a meaningful and healthy way (and yes, we certainly can do this), we will keep in mind certain considerations.

We will, for instance, take care to distinguish between *trauma* and how grief or shame or PTSD expresses vs. *dysautonomia* and how a dysregulated nervous system presents. Most patients will come to the clinical encounter with a level of emotional trauma and it may or may not be part of their narrative in the treatment room. This is not the same as having a nervous system that jolts in terror for no reason or relentless anxiety. As practitioners of Chinese medicine, we are more inclined to read this situation for what it is if we ponder it. When we draw direct connections between the patient's organs and emotions without assigning meaning to the emotional states, we are addressing the dysregulated nervous system in the way that it needs to be treated. It is when we start bringing metaphysical value judgements into the clinical assessment that we are no longer addressing the root cause of the patient's ostensible psychological suffering.[11]

A hyper-reactive autonomic nervous system coupled with

intestines that do not move properly may be diagnosed by the MD as anxiety. But is it? It could be that the person's body, independent of trauma, is unable to regulate their adrenaline. When we treat for anxiety, depression, PTSD, extremes of grief, or anything that could fit within the rubric of Liver qi stagnation, shen disturbance, Heart Heat leading to mania, or other similar, we factor in the way an EDS body might contain a hyper-reactive autonomic nervous system just because—apart from anything psycho-emotional—the effects of HCTDs on the nervous system are often substantive. Identifying what could be attributed to a manifestation of the patient's connective tissue snarled by a hyper-reactive autonomic nervous system vs. the patient's expression of, say, PTSD or other trauma is something that a practitioner must do if they wish to adequately address the issues at hand.

There is a lot that we can do for patients without becoming a de facto psychotherapist. People with EDS tend to have higher levels of anxiety and more neurological differences such as ADHD and autism or autism spectrum. Most patients want to relieve their anxiety and are satisfied if this occurs as a result of their acupuncture treatment. Some want to stop taking Ritalin or other drugs commonly given for attention disorder. Others do not. Either way, it helps them if the practitioner can calm their shen. There is a large neurodivergent community spread across social media with the result that autistic persons are becoming less isolated and more supported in their identities. A patient is under no obligation to make any adjustment to their divergence but, by treating the shen, we are able to support their wellbeing and sense of calm.[12]

Compare, for instance, two of my patients with chronic and deeply held emotional injury.

The first, a woman, had been diagnosed with hEDS. Her childhood was marked by severe abuse. She developed a prolapsed uterus, bladder, and rectum, for which she underwent surgical revision. Her ankles and feet were painful and her joints alternated between being extremely, frighteningly loose and painfully, excruciatingly tight. Her medical team was extensive. She came to me for treatment of chronic pain and if the subject of emotional injury came up, she became agitated. She did not want to change her diet unless her nutritionist directed her to do so, and she was drug sensitive and would not take calming formulas or any such medication not prescribed by her psychiatrist.

I could have treated this as a case of shen disturbance, Heart–Kidney disharmony, or Liver qi stagnation. From my perspective as a practitioner of Chinese medicine, there was a lot that I could do for her psyche that would then affect her physical body. Instead, I focused solely on Bi syndrome and remained within the realm that she afforded me. Yes, I put seeds or needles in the shenmen points of her ears and soothed via yintang and other relevant points. She also felt less anxious when she experienced a reduction in her pain, so indirectly, I did address emotional wellbeing. This patient had multiple concerns and felt safer under the care of her psychologist and psychiatrist. By reducing pain, we made it probable that her work with her team would be successful. That was the safest approach and that is what we did.

Another patient was the opposite. He, too, had psycho-emotional issues that left marks on his mind and body. This patient came to me for treatment of erectile dysfunction. Over time, it became clear that hEDS or HSD was a potential factor. This patient did not want to work on pain, even though his discomfort within his body was pressing. Instead, "being stressed" was something that he understood. Focusing on the goal of calming the shen and soothing the Liver (aka "resolving stress") made sense to him and he went along with the program until we had a successful outcome with respect to his initial complaint (attributed to Kidney yang deficiency and Cold). As he felt a greater sense of efficacy with one part of his body, it became easier to accept the idea that he might want to see a rheumatologist. Not right at the moment, but the seed was planted for when he was ready.

Trauma is a culturally mediated experience. How the law responds to trauma, the way it is handled at the doctor's office, its story within diagnostic manuals, and the cultural narratives that contain it all have a role in how trauma expresses in mind, body, and spirit. EDS is a disorder of connective tissue, and connective tissue runs throughout the entire body. There is nothing untouched by connective tissue. The hydra, in psycho-emotional terrains, is as slippery and untouchable as it will be, whether or not the outcomes of it are dire or barely noticeable. As long as we are aware of our own boundaries, and the boundaries that our patients need to maintain, we have valuable tools within our medical tradition with which to calm the shen and nurture a healthy spirit.

## Gu Syndrome

We are often a last resort for patients with mysterious diseases. They may have done everything and, in desperation, they think it wouldn't hurt to at least "try acupuncture." They may have been given pharmaceutical drugs that, technically, "work" but which left them so ill from side effects that the net gain was negligible and the patient went right back to square one. Undiagnosed hEDS patients are often categorized as having medically uncertain symptoms (MUS). Most of us have had patients with mold toxicity or chronic illness following Lyme disease. Long-haul COVID sufferers and, increasingly, those deemed histamine intolerant, if not frankly suffering from MCAS, are also mystery-illness patients we serve. Gu syndrome is not altogether out of line when considering which pattern applies to these patients, especially if we refocus our lens and place this ancient theory of illness in a contemporary context.

But what does this term mean? How does it (does it?) translate to modern medicine? If it does, how can it be connected with hereditary illness? There is an entry for Gu toxin in *A Practical Dictionary of Chinese Medicine* and I replicate it in full, "Ancient disease name denoting various severe conditions that have been equated with scrub typhus, chronic blood fluke infestation, severe hepatitis, cirrhosis of the liver, and severe bacillary or amebic dysentery of modern medicine" (Wiseman and Feng 1998, p.250). This description posits the term as archaic. However, the diseases its parameters encompass are known, accepted, and addressed by modern medicine. The entry does not give much useful information regarding the overarching reach of Gu syndrome.[13]

If we apply a working notion of Gu syndrome to treatment of patients with Lyme disease, mold toxicity, and/or chronic and indeterminate disease, it is instructive to reference German-born and American-based classical scholar and practitioner, Heiner Fruehauf. According to Fruehauf, the character which denotes Gu refers to debilitating chronic parasite infection (2008, p.1). Translating this condition to contemporary time shifts the narrative. Indeed, "[current] definition of Gu syndrome points to aggressive helminthic, protozoan, fungal spirochete, or viral afflictions that have become systemic in an immune compromised patient" (*ibid.*, p.1). Of his clinical experience treating Lyme patients, Fruehauf declares that, "I can say with great certainty that, from a classical Chinese perspective, Lyme is a specific type of Gu Syndrome" (2011a, p.20).

As a practitioner of Chinese medicine trained in the United States, my knowledge of Gu syndrome (gu zheng) was limited to hearing occasional references made by instructors in my program. I was not formally taught about it during coursework. As my practice has grown and my experience treating hEDS and MCAS has increased, I have returned to the classics of Chinese medicine in order to construct a greater understanding of its foundations. Though I might be disinclined to specifically identify a syndrome by the term Gu, I do see the same elements (Damp and Phlegm, especially) in the patterns I see in certain patients.

Translations can be enlightening. Medical literature from centuries gone by paints an evocative scenario; we visualize, for instance, the description in *Raising the Dead and Returning Life: Emergency Medicine in the Qing Dynasty* by Bao Xiang'áo, of a patient who suffered from what he calls a "harm-striking spirit" type of Gu. The Qing-era physician's case report explains that, "[the patient's] spirit is clouded, his temperament is agitated, his eyes see evil ghost shapes, his ears hear evil ghost sounds. He acts as if he has committed a felony, as if there were armed soldiers pursuing him..." (2012, p.148). Something is inside this patient that has overtaken him, and he suffers. Herbs that we know, today, will help him; "The formula to treat this," the physician wrote, "is modified Chai Hu Tang" (*ibid.*, p.148). The patient must also adhere to a healing diet.

Descriptions of Gu syndrome resonate. Even if our patients are not quite as tormented as those described by the Qing-dynasty practitioner, if we have had patients with chronic night terrors, for instance, or intractable anxiety, we will agree that their stories are similar. Yet the push to modernize and become integrative by adapting to Western biomedicine's precepts has not been favorable to the notion of Gu, and Freuhauf notes that, "mainland Chinese scholars generally dismiss it as an 'ancient, feudalist and superstitious' belief in demons and exorcist practices that has little or no value in modern clinical practice" (1998, p.1).

Still, the question remains: what can a practitioner do when a patient is suffering from a collection of symptoms that defy biomedical diagnosis? We routinely engage with complicated presentations and chronic disease, but hEDS plus Lyme or mold toxicity or MCAS is a different beast entirely. Might we look through the lens of Gu syndrome when the patient is afflicted by deeply held pathogens that biomedicine will identify as, "systemic fungal infection (primarily candidiasis), systemic parasite infection, chronic viral infection, or a combination thereof" (*ibid.*, p.9)? We may choose not to rely entirely on the Gu narrative, but we certainly can use it as a starting point and a touchstone for critical thinking.

A contemporary reconstruction of Gu syndrome encompasses two manifestations, one of which pertains to gut health and another that is reflected in the neurological realm. Fruehauf describes "Digestive Gu" as a compendium of bloating, gas, and/or difficulty with bowel movement such as IBS, all of which is exacerbated by brain fog, chronic fatigue, and perhaps strange dreams. His description of "Brain Gu" fixes this presentation in the neurological realm and he describes patients with chronic pain, headache, depression, anxiety, and/or hallucinations. Fruehauf explains the challenging, pervasive nature of this illness by referring to ancient sources, noting that, "it says clearly in the classical texts that the nature of Gu syndrome can be compared to oil seeping into flour. This is much different from a pearl falling into flour—with a pearl, you can just take tweezers and remove it" (2008, p.8).

Classical Chinese texts described Gu as worms in a pot, and brain Gu, Fruehauf explains, is set in motion by, "chronic viruses that target the nervous system (such as coxsackie, herpes, and in some cases HIV), or spirochetes (especially Lyme and its coinfections), or other exotic pathogens causing chronic forms of meningitis, malaria, leptospirosis, etc." and he includes patients diagnosed with fibromyalgia within this profile (*ibid.*, p.19). Fruehauf argues that Gu today entails, "digestive distress, coupled with neurological distress, such as body pain or mental symptoms—light symptoms such as fogginess, or severe symptoms such as hallucinations—that [is] not explainable with Western medicine, and that [is] not explainable either by regular diagnostic patterning that we learned in TCM school" (*ibid.*, p.15). While the original link of Gu to demonic possession no longer applies to contemporary medical theory, certainly the signs and symptoms that prevail do.[14]

There is tremendous potential in working either from the perspective of Gu, the psyche, the Earth center, and/or the physical body in pain. We consider the patient's bigger picture and the team they have in place (or not). We pay attention to where the patient is and what they are ready to tackle. We never rush. Everything in its time and place.

In so doing, we provide an invaluable resource to a deserving patient population.


## III. Low and Slow: Thoughts on Herbal Medicine


A perennial question in EDS support groups runs along the lines of, "Do you respond normally to pharma drugs?" I find the responses affirming. People often relate anecdotes that resonate with my own experience, both personally and in my clinic. There are always a few who say that they cannot take anything.

My answer is that if there are any rare adverse events possible when taking a pharma drug, I will experience them. I will say that if it were not for Chinese medicine, I would have no medicine at all. I share this not to center myself, to be clear. Instead, I do so to clarify my subjectivity. This is not a matter of reading the studies or finding data to support a hypothesis, though these do exist.[15] It is my lived experience. It is nice that research studies show that being drug sensitive exists. But I have felt less alone and much more affirmed by reading responses in social media groups that mirror what I know to be true. To wit: some of us really, truly are the canaries in the coal mines of pharmaceutical intervention.[16]

A person with any HCTD will have specific concerns when deciding whether or not to take medication. Whether or not and how to prescribe herbal formulas for patients is more a matter of, "What kind of patient is this?" than, "Which syndrome is this and what is the treatment principle?" At least at first, anyway. A practitioner of Chinese medicine will also need to keep not only the patients and their potentially volatile metabolisms in mind, but also their context. As per the first section of this chapter, there are types of patients (diagnosed or not; searching for answers to their medical mystery vs. oblivious). Where they fit on this spectrum will determine whether to prescribe herbs, what to consider prescribing, and how to do so safely and effectively.

Most diagnosed patients know the drill. When patients already have been up and down the EDS mountain a few times and they know that the practitioner already has done the same, the need to elaborate beyond a simple declaration ("I am extremely drug sensitive and react bizarrely to everything") is minimal. When a patient knows that the practitioner understands, the patient is more trusting and willing to try herbal formulas. Being able to speak the language of histamine intolerance and demonstrating awareness of MCAS is also reassuring to patients, no matter what categories define their subject position. If a practitioner does not have a dedicated practice in support of HCTDs, the patient may be anxious about herbal medicine and less inclined to try it.

A practitioner will consider whether or not the patient is diagnosed and working with a large medical team vs. diagnosed or self-diagnosed and not working with allopathic providers. The needs of these individuals will differ from those of our undiagnosed patients who look to Chinese medicine because they want answers to their medical mysteries. This is not the same as the patient who comes in for something entirely different, completely unaware that the flexibility that is normal to them might not actually be within a normative frame to support health. Within all of these categories resides the question of adverse event history. Some patients, diagnosed or not, there for HCTD treatment or obliviously at the clinic for something else, will have a known history of poor reactions to drugs. Others will say that they are allergic to penicillin, but this is because patients are trained by the medical system to identify such an allergy.

People are not necessarily trained to know things like what constitutes a history of unwarranted reactivity to medication. If it is "normal" to feel poorly after a certain vaccine or pill, at what point does this become a pattern that is cause for concern? A practitioner needs to become expert at asking the questions that elicit the information we need in order to provide safe prescriptions. Intake forms ask for allergies to drugs but if we treat HCTD patients, we must be more specific. Asking a patient to talk about what has happened when they have taken an antifungal or if they have any stories about not reacting well to local anesthesia can uncover meaningful information. *In what way* does the patient respond poorly to the combination of lidocaine and epinephrine that is commonly used by dentists to block pain during procedures? *What happened* when they took an antibiotic?

The question is not, "Did you have an adverse reaction?" because patients may have had adverse reactions to a number of drugs but been gaslit and told that what they experienced was not serious. This teaches people to ignore their bodies and to not trust their own perceptions. It also sets them up for even worse adverse events if the extreme reaction compounds. Instead of inquiring about adverse reactions, we can ask, "What happened when you took…?" If the answers begin to show a pattern, then this is a patient who needs a conservative approach with herbal medicine. An excellent guide can be found in the work of Qin Bo-Wei, whose training and philosophy privileged gentle formulas and clear, simple treatment principles. The translated *Qin Bo-Wei's 56 Treatment Methods: Writing Precise Prescriptions* (Wu 2011) is an invaluable resource for a practitioner who works with medication-sensitive patients.

I will also take this moment to share a personal anecdote.

Leaving aside my history of reacting badly to every pharma

drug I have ever taken, and not wasting time telling stories about how I react to anesthesia at the dentist, it suffices to share an anecdote regarding a minor surgery that required stitches. Years ago, I had a skin growth that my PCP wanted to remove. She gave me an injection to numb the area but when she began to cut, I felt all of it. I asked, in a reasonably calm voice, how long it would take to finish and said, apologetically, that I did not think the shot had worked. My doctor stopped, and when I said that I could tolerate it if I knew how long things would take, she protested, saying that she was not going to give me stitches if I could feel them. She was quite upset on my behalf. I said, "Ok, just give me a moment." Her assistant was next to the exam table to my left, so I leaned my forehead into the crook of their arm and wheezed. I allowed myself to indulge in one small panic attack, and then I turned back to my doctor and said, "Ok, I'm fine, go ahead."

Both my doctor and the assistant stared at me with their mouths hanging open in shock. My doctor said, "You are so tough, my God. Most patients would be screaming and you're so docile." She and the assistant both marveled and agreed that most patients would have reacted far differently.

I did not have the heart to tell her that the second shot, though more effective than the first, wore off quickly and that I did feel the stitches. I left the office feeling gratified by the way they marveled at my toughness (I am tough and I am proud of it) but I also experienced a profound sense of shame. This doesn't happen to normal people, I thought, and I wondered what was wrong with me. I cried a little bit when I got to my car, because it was painful and I felt stupid and like a freak. Then I drove home and forgot it until, years later, I learned about hEDS and how there are people who do not react as expected to pharmaceutical drugs, including anesthetics. This is a cautionary tale for any medical care practitioner. Some patients honestly do not know that what they experience is unusual or that it warrants extra attention.

Asking about drug history if the person doesn't have the knowledge or perspective to determine that no, really, this or that reaction is part of a larger response pattern that needs to be noted requires questions that actually elicit the desired information. "What happened when you took [X drug]?" is much more useful than, "Have you ever reacted badly to any drugs?"

If the individual's pre-Heaven essence constructed them in a unique way, then we as practitioners need to be aware that reactions to herbal formulas might express in an equally unique manner. A patient with vEDS will most likely know that this is their subtype, but this is not always so, and these are patients who need to be extraordinarily careful with any Blood-moving herbs because they are vulnerable to aortic dissection and cardiac events.[17] A patient with MCAS might have an extreme reaction that makes no sense whatsoever, but they have it, or they may respond well one day and have a ghastly overreaction the next. There is a reason why the phrase "low and slow" is popular in chronic illness communities. A person is safest when they start with a low dose and smartest to move slowly with any increases or changes.

A person who is diagnosed may not want to try herbal medicine. Their allopathic team might not want them to try herbal medicine. Eventually, though, they may decide that they want to stop taking pharma drugs. It is ethical to be encouraging and supportive and it is wise to have the patient make the shift under their MD's supervision. Pharma drugs have a level of built-in protection from charges of being unsafe or unregulated or potentially harmful. This may not be warranted, but the structures supporting the biomedical industrial complex, Big Pharma as an entity, and narratives surrounding standard of care all protect a pharma adverse event more readily than an herbal one. This patient population may not react as expected and it is best to unambiguously maintain the boundary between the pharmaceutical intervention and the herbal. It is wise to clearly leave the responsibility for outcomes of pharma drugs to the biomedical physician of record. Once the patient is successfully weaned off the anti-anxiety or antidepressant medication (or the low-dose naltrexone or whatever) and the MD clears them from taking the drug further, then we can begin a course of herbal medicine.

Aside from the matter of drug sensitivity, there are HCTD considerations that factor into herbal strategies. Esophageal spasm history and/or an unstable cervical spine means that a larger tablet might be hard for the patient to swallow. Raw herbs are wonderful but if the patient is exhausted by chronic pain, they will not have the energy to brew herbal tea. Accessibility and ease of use are important. Tea pills, tinctures, or powder are better for these patients.

I consider two of my favorite formulas here, and share an adjacent one that may be a good substitute. Most of us know these formulas and do not need extensive commentary; consequently, my remarks accompanying them are brief and confined to how they relate to hEDS. I do not include dosage because each patient is unique and the practitioner will determine what is safe in each instance.

Bu Zhong Yi Qi Tang (BZYQT) is Li Dong-Yuan's most famous formula and it is commonly used in the treatment of three patterns: Spleen and Stomach deficiency, qi deficiency fever, and qi sinking in the middle Jiao. All three of these patterns can be common in an hEDS presentation. Its chief herb, *Huang Qi*, generally tends to be safe for people with hEDS and, though termed Astragalus by individuals not familiar with Chinese medicine, it is an herb familiar to many in chronic illness communities. If the patient is concerned about taking an unknown herb, we can reassure them by using the English-language term. If the practitioner is concerned about MCAS hyper-reactivity, it is possible to ask them if they have tried Astragalus and how they responded. This is an excellent formula, not only due to its efficacy but also because its main component is something that hEDS patients may know or already have tried.

The concept of yin Fire in contemporary medicine is not entirely stable but it resonates when one is familiar with HCTDs. Scheid *et al.* point out that there is ambiguity in the original text associated with Li Dong-Yuan and enough scholarly dissent regarding meaning that, "these discussions will never truly be closed" (2009, p.319). My clinical experience with dysautonomia, especially, makes the notion of yin Fire intriguing. BZYQT, "is, above all, a formula for the treatment of fevers that arise from a dysfunction of the yin and yang organs in the interior or yin aspect of the body, and not from the penetration of pathogenic cold into the exterior or yang aspect of the body" (*ibid.*, p.319). Patients who tend to be very cold, as is common with hEDS patients, will also experience, "yang symptoms such as... headache, dizziness, palpitations, tinnitus...and..., fever will be accompanied by sweating and aversion to cold; headache is aggravated by exertion, etc." (*ibid.*, p.319). There are dysautonomia presentations that will express in the way described here.

A less-ambiguous impetus for relying on BZYQT is the matter of prolapse and/or ptosis. Scheid *et al.* list the biomedical indications for this formula, including, "those related to a slackening of muscles or other tissues such as uterine prolapse, prolapsed rectum, gastroptosis, hernias, stress incontinence, myasthenia gravis, primary hypotension, and constipation due to decreased peristalsis" (*ibid.*, p.321). In other words, the extremely common comorbid conditions that an hEDS specialist will treat. For chronic pain, BZYQT can be modified by the addition of *Xi Xin*, and pronounced Cold can be ameliorated by the inclusion of *Rou Gui* (*ibid.*, p.322).

Interestingly, there is commentary in *56 Treatment Methods* that specifically mentions yin Fire as being less common in the modern day. Drs. Qin and Wu state that they only saw a true yin Fire presentation in severely Spleen qi deficient patients (Wu

2011, p.75). Given that the so-called rare disease that is hEDS is often a matter of the patient being severely Spleen qi deficient, this resonates. I only have seen what I view as yin Fire in my hEDS patients. They further note that the relationship of prolapse to Spleen qi sinking has become more apparent when treating contemporary patients than it was before, simply because modern imaging tools make it easier to diagnose ptosis and prolapse (Wu 2011, p.76). A practitioner who specializes in hEDS treatment will become familiar with yin Fire and prolapse. BZYQT is also useful for erectile dysfunction patients with hEDS who do not respond to testosterone therapy.

How I understood the *Pi Wei Lun* ten years ago compared with how I read it now is akin to the difference between reading *Don Quijote* as a teenager vs. reviewing it over and over and over again for my Ph.D. qualifying exams. This is a text worthy of multiple translations and, ideally, copious annotation. A practitioner must maintain the hope that the work of this venerable ancestor will one day be revisited by current generations of translators. Though Chinese medicine does not have a specific diagnosis of EDS, it is clear that ancient physicians saw not only patients exhausted by overwork and poor diet but, too, they treated people with connective tissue disorder. Pondering the theories of Li Gao brings us closer to understanding our patients' complex presentations. And, while BZYQT is a worthy formula for hEDS patients, it is not a cure and the practitioner will likely need to modify it. Still, the fact that Astragalus is a known herb in EDS communities and that it is a formula seemingly created for these populations means that a practitioner can begin here with confidence.

Prolapse, of course, is not the only hallmark of hEDS that we will see in our clinics. MCAS is another ubiquitous challenge. Yin Qiao San (YQS), for its part, is my favorite formula. Though the actions of YQS respond to upper respiratory infection with Heat signs, my experience is that it is also useful in response to MCAS. In fact, YQS is my most trusted and beloved formula for what may be called, if we are speaking from the perspective of Chinese medicine, rebellious wei qi or, perhaps more properly in some manifestations of it, Wind. Interestingly, the use of antihistamines to treat anxiety and depression is gaining traction in Western biomedicine and I have had hEDS patients who were prescribed them for this purpose.[18] Dialing down a hyper-reactive immune system can be calming, and YQS in some cases can do just this.

We might also consider a similar formula, Shuang Huang Lian (SHL). My preference is always for the former. However, the latter has been studied for its efficacy in addressing MCAS. The choice to use one or the other may rest on the patient's contextual factors. If the patient's MD does not support them taking herbal medicine, it can be easier to prescribe SHL and to send the patient a link to the Yuan Gao *et al.* article, "The three-herb formula Shuang-Huang-Lian stabilizes mast cells through activation of mitochondrial calcium uniporter."[19] This way, the MD can see that there is research behind the choice. Otherwise, my clinical and personal experience with YQS is that it can be exceptionally useful, especially for skin-related presentations.

Any herbal formula can be efficacious and safe if the prescription has been filtered through the unique needs of the individual patient with dysfunctional connective tissue. As with anything that we do, we base our decisions on what is normal for an HCTD body and what is necessary for its safety. Connective tissue is an element of the vascular system, and the patient's blood might be disordered, so we are mindful with Blood-moving herbs. We take into account that MCAS can be serious and we start slowly. We pay attention to the patient who says that they are drug sensitive and we learn to ask the right questions to elicit meaningful information in case the patient is not sure what that really means.

All of the above caveats aside, it is also necessary to remember how genuinely life-changing Chinese herbal medicine can be for hypersensitive patients. It is exciting to see how herbs can radically improve a patient's health. With some folks, it barely takes anything to see marked improvement. And for others, Chinese herbal medicine will be the only medicine that they can take. Indeed, Chinese herbal medicine can be a lifesaver. When we start low and go slow, it is amazing what we can do for our patients.

# CHAPTER 4

# Getting to the Point

## I. Readings in Translation: The Tangible Body

Diagnosis pulls from the distant past. It gathers the here and now into an exchange between practitioner and patient in a tangible space: the clinical encounter. The tangible body finds its center in the process of naming its condition. My narrative in *Chinese Medicine* follows the same path, touching now on what is palpable: the body. I begin by considering historical views; speaking to translations that engage with bodies, I question received wisdom on this very subject. The center of this chapter presents a tour of organs and channels as viewed through the filter of HCTD. Whether we begin our treatment strategy by starting with the channels, organs, or point prescriptions is contingent, and fluid; consequently, I focus on the *where* of treatment here, leaving the *how* of modality to chapter five. Finally, I return to the body's inner wrappings. Before the subsequent chapter and its discussion of methods, I review ideas regarding another important tissue—the fascia—and place this material within a larger context of channel theory.

How anyone might view a body is mediated by a multitude of filters both personal and professional. These include languages, cultures, ways of knowing, and medicine's stories, whether Chinese or other. When one's own body is constructed by tissue that deviates from what is considered the norm, that is one thing.

Quite another is to be charged with tending to such bodies and to discerning whether that body might become healthier, this one may not, and the next has potential but might never be quite as vigorous or stable as its owner might wish. To read the body is to embody the filters of one's medical profession. This viewing depends on the lessons from our medical forebears who shape our vision. Connective tissue disorder, for its part, asks us to revisit how Chinese medicine views the tangible body.

Beginning with historical perspective, we reflect upon classical conceptions of the human form. Shigehisa Kuriyama's elegant assessment of differences between Asian and Occidental perspectives, *The Expressiveness of the Body and the Divergence of Greek and Chinese Medicine*, references the West's Plato, Galen, and muscles as compared to pulse and breath in China. His argument holds that an absence of focus on the muscular body is a key aspect in the development of Asian medicine. Kuriyama sees in these differences the root of contemporary divergence, noting that, "This is how conceptions of the body diverge – not just in the meanings that each ascribes to bodily signs, but more fundamentally in the changes and features that each recognizes as signs" (1999, p.272). He posits that musculature, which characterizes Western depictions of the body, did not factor into classical Chinese portrayals of the human form, thus placing certain filters over perception and ways of knowing that persist, to a certain degree, even unto today.

I would have found this book interesting as a humanities professor. I would have deemed it persuasive. Indeed, it is both. As a former humanities professor and current practitioner of Chinese medicine, I am also inclined to delve deeper into the narrative of my own lived practice. I do not believe that ancient Chinese physicians overlooked the body to the extent that scholar-physicians of that time might have implied that they did. I wish I could read classical Chinese and verify this through my own meticulous reading of original and source texts, but that is not available to me. In Spanish literature, though, we would look to something called *lo nimio* if we were searching for the small everyday details that spoke the heart of the people. This term means something small or insignificant, and when I consider it in relation to literature, usually I think of the poet Antonio Machado, who wrote about the Spanish countryside and the humble folk who were the soul of his cherished country.[1]

Though not examples of classical literature, per se, I will in the context of Chinese medicine instead refer to two translations by scholar and practitioner Lorraine Wilcox. They are instructive. Both *Categorized Essentials of Repairing the Body Zhèng Ti Lèi Yào* and *Raising the Dead and Returning Life: Emergency Medicine in the Qing Dynasty* are, as their titles suggest, practical texts reflective of physicians who dealt with bodies in pain. In the first, we learn how a practitioner during the Ming-dynasty period resolves broken bones and other serious injuries. In the second, we discover the first aid practices of common people in South China during the mid-nineteenth century.

This is not the noble medicine of a Zhang Zhongjing or a Sun Si Miao or a Hua Tuo. Instead, the books describe maladies resulting from traumatic injury, ranging from beatings and canings to hangings and falls from a horse. These are wounds caused by blows from life itself.

The preface to *Categorized Essentials* begins with a lament over the way in which repairing the body (in essence, traumatology) is not recognized in Chinese medicine. The preface's author, Lù Shīdào, asks a rhetorical question, "Isn't the skill of rejoining and restoring [sinews and bones] displayed in the subtlety of manual techniques?" His answer, which may resonate with modern-day tui na practitioners, is resigned and telling, "But the labor of pressing and probing is scorned as unskilled work, so no one discusses it" (Xuē 2017, p.24). At least, this resonated with me as I remembered the period right after I was granted my license to practice acupuncture. "Are you still going to practice tui na?"

was a question I heard more than once; when I replied in the affirmative, the response was often, "Why would you do that?"[2]

"Pressing and probing" is not unskilled work, especially if one's patient population suffers from connective tissue disorder and, as one who does just so, I read this book with great interest. There are clinical pearls within it that correspond with what I have determined empirically. "If the bones and sockets have been rejoined but repeatedly dislocate, the liver and kidneys are deficient" writes Dr. Xuē (*ibid.*, p.32). In his time, this was a reference to green swellings that do not ulcerate and, though this is of course not something I see in my clinic, it is also true that hEDS joints that repeatedly separate do so based on patterns related to Liver and Kidney deficiency. I have patients who fit this description.

Later in the text, I read with great interest the case of Official Yáng who dislocated a bone. Though it was reinserted into the joint, the patient continued to suffer pain due to what Dr. Xuē perceived to be Liver Fire. In response, the good physician started his patient on a course of modified Xiao Chai Hu Tang (XCHT) and subsequently dosed him with Si Wu Tang (SWT) modified with *Zhi Zi*, *Huang Bai*, and *Zhi Mu*. Fortunately, Official Yáng, "took proper care of himself and became healthy" (*ibid.*, p.77).

We recollect that in the thirteenth chapter of the *Ling Shu* there is discussion pertaining to the sinews. The description outlines the geography of this tissue, the symptoms that the sinews evince when in distress, and the ways in which a practitioner might address dysfunction. The chapter concludes with a concise description of the effects of temperature (Cold and Hot) on the sinews that is reflected in the above-mentioned report regarding Official Yáng. The chapter clearly shows that physicians of the time period viewed the dysfunction caused by contracted or flaccid sinews as worthy of note. Further, if we wish to view an hEDS presentation through this lens, we will note that, according the *Nei Jing*, Cold will result in contracture while Heat, on the other hand, makes the tendons loose. This declaration, especially if taken in the context of Li Dong-Yuan's observations on the nature of yin Fire, are salient to the matter of HCTD and hEDS.

We have our narratives from venerable medical ancestors and we compare them to stories told today. Contemporary biomedicine, for its part, is incredibly eager to find a specific genetic mutation that is the cause of hEDS. Connective tissue disorder can be serious and life-threatening; finding a specific gene is viewed as the first step in treatment strategy. It also validates the suffering of the patient. There is a something that can be objectively seen and thus, in turn, a door is opened to proper treatment and, one hopes, one day a cure. So very much hinges on the notion of finding a genetic link, a visible (though not tangible) something that says, "Here it is, right here. The disorder exists and the patient has it."

The role of the gene in conferring validity and a point of departure for healthcare strategies is an intriguing topic for anyone who enjoys tracing the development of thought and scientific advance. It is quite fascinating to look at the third edition of McKusick's *Heritable Disorders of Connective Tissue* (the earliest one I could acquire, which was a banged-up old library copy from Ohio University). Published in 1966, it consists of detailed descriptions and photographs of suffering patients, many of them in their underwear. Some are naked. Most are set in front of a white background like criminals in an old-fashioned police line-up. The next copy of this text that I purchased was the fifth edition, which was edited by Peter Beighton. Now, or at least at the now of the fifth edition, in 1993, researchers had well and truly become fluent in genomics science. Now, half the book consists of the photographs and detailed narratives provided by Dr. McKusick; much of the text, now, is couched in the knowledge of discoveries that were not available until thirty or so years ago.

The contrast, as one goes along reading the volume, between the photographs from the original volume and the newest genetic excitement evinced by the second half of the text, makes the book feel, in an odd sort of way, disjointed. What is accepted now will be undone soon enough. Even as I wrote *Chinese Medicine*, new information made itself available for anyone who wanted to look for it.[3]

We learn by acquiring, by testing, by contesting. We learn by comparison. The practitioner of Chinese medicine who is unable to access original texts may feel somewhat disjointed after their own fashion. Someone who does not speak Chinese and who lacks the skill to read classical Chinese is constrained by the skill of translators and the ability to find translated works. We owe translators a tremendous debt of gratitude for their work. And while a practitioner like Dr. Xuē might not enjoy the approbation of a Hua Tuo, there is no doubt that he was concerned with the way muscle attached to bone and the interchange between bone and ligament. Nobody who tends to bodies that have been caned could do otherwise. We may need to look a little harder to find these practitioners, especially if we do not speak the language, but they existed. Their patients' joints healed because they were treated with knowledge and care.[4]

Interest in the tangible body can also be seen in the work of Wang Qing-ren, a practitioner who argued for a review of anatomy in the early nineteenth century. The physician himself claimed to study the bodies of deceased children and condemned criminals in order to study in great detail the inner working of the human form. That his work was, to a large degree, erroneous does not discount his contributions to the subject of Blood stasis. His impassioned argument does mention errors in perception of the sinew channels and his missive is driven by an urge to challenge received wisdom and expand the horizons of his professional peers. That his legacy is primarily within the realm of herbal formulas to correct Blood stasis does not lessen the value of his attempts to challenge his antecedents.[5]

Neither Dr. Ehlers nor Dr. Danlos was looking for the collagen disorders when they found the patients who brought them everlasting fame. They were dermatologists who studied syphilis. Though Peter and Greta Beighton's lively biographical sketches of physicians who have syndromes that now bear their names, including the aforementioned two doctors, describe their lives and legacies, I have been unable to trace the thread from syphilis to lax connective tissue.[6] One has to wonder what they were looking for when they found what is now their eponymous syndrome.

As we look back to our medical ancestors and parse their views on what aspects of the body are more important and which aspects of health and disease merit attention, it may well be that, back then, "the labor of pressing and probing is scorned as unskilled work, so no one discusses it" (Xuē 2017, p.24). Consequently, what survived in the literary legacy reflects what is not scorned. It is fancier to be able to look at a patient and just know, I guess, and exceptional pulse-taking skill followed by an even more phenomenal ability to write an herbal prescription will always confer value to the practitioner. Then and now, privilege is as privilege does. But we may sift through the literature, albeit in translation, and we may look to resources pertaining to tui na and to the art of palpation, and we will find what we seek. The sinews are full of stories and they speak, I think, most clearly to hands that know how to listen. There are pearls to be discovered regarding joints and tissues and the soul that these substances contain if we know where to look, even in translation, within the extant historical record.

## II. Organs and Channels, from Top to Toe

### Taiyin Channel and Organs

Viewing the body as a geographical expanse is telling in the case of the Lung and the Spleen channels. Any interpretation of hEDS will more than likely begin and end with the Spleen organ. Either approach—organ first, channel second or vice versa—would work, but in my estimation, it is the channel, or the geography of the body, that tells us more of what we want to know. Besides, the channels draw us inward, ultimately, towards the organs. Though we may opt to consider the organs from a classical perspective, we are not fixed into a singular perspective.[7] The Lung pertains to the skin, as we know, while the Spleen pertains to flesh. The two systems, Lung and Spleen, belong to the one channel, taiyin of the hand and foot, and how they can be read according to the needs of hEDS constitutes the focus of this section.

There are touchstones that characterize the Lung, whether or not there is an hEDS body containing it. As we know, the Lung is the yang within yin organ. It is a canopy. This organ, with its in and out breath, is our interface with the external world. What damages the Lung include external factors such as Wind, Heat, Cold and internal factors such as grief. What is taken in and what is expelled have their processes, as we know. The Lung's paired organ is the Large Intestine and, in that relationship, we can trace the taking in of a pure nutrient (air) and the expulsion of what is no longer needed (waste). The color associated with the Lung is white, its element is metal, and of the spiritual aspect, the Lung is associated with the po, or spirit-mind that comes to life with the Lung's first breath and departs with its last.

A body whose connective tissue betrays it may not breathe easily due not to the Kidneys' failure to grasp qi nor to deficiency in the Lung itself. Instead, loose ribs and inflamed cartilage might make the physical act of inspiration a punishment. We might hear from our patients that they have icy cold hands and feet and that, though not diabetic, they constantly need to urinate and that, when they do, the urine is copious and clear. The Lung's relation to Kidney is evident in such a presentation and it may be, barring the matter of dysautonomia, the aforementioned failure to grasp the qi. In my experience, structural defect (weak or tight ribs) and the Lung–Kidney relationship are the most common root causes of Lung dysfunction in my hEDS patients. It may well be, too, that the issue at hand pertains to grief.

One of my favorite points is LU-3. Tianfu, or Palace of Heaven, is a Window of Heaven point. On a pragmatic level, it is useful for purple-white blotches (pityriasis versicolor), which is common with hEDS. I also have seen how it frames grief. In *Explanations of Channels and Points*, we find in Yuè Hánzhēn's commentary on LU-4 a clinical pearl. Regarding Heart pain, the sage reminds that, "the lung is metal; the heart is fire" and notes the significance of pain plus a deficient left cun pulse. He says, "This is the wife exploiting the position of the husband; therefore, seek this point [i.e., LU-4] in order to sooth lung qì, to prevent it from interfering with the heart" (2019, p.15). When I feel a deficient left cun pulse, I ask the patient if they have allergies or, if not, whether they have been crying. If the patient has cried recently, then I am never surprised when I palpate and find coldness between LU-3 and 4 and a divot in this Window of Heaven point.

Is this indicative of the Heart's joy conflicting with the Lung's relationship to grief? Soothing the qi via LU-3 seems to restore a sense of balance and calm to patients, and this is true of many, not just my hEDS patients. However, what is striking in the latter cases is the coldness of this point in combination with a deficient left cun pulse.

Grief and flow of qi if we are starting from the perspective of treating the shen can center on LU-3; moving to LU-6, we might opt to treat acute pain and stiffness. Chronic pain tends to be systematic, but ebbs and flows of new discomforts and the danger when one subluxes a joint are acute issues that plague these patients. Though LU-5 is an exceptional point for many reasons, it is wise to be careful when needling directly over joints. Some patients are fragile and it is prudent to find adjacent points, either up- or downstream, rather than getting too close to the joints. LU-7 is another example of this caution. As I elucidate in chapter five, these are points that can often be treated via ear seeds. In order to avoid disruption to the stability of the connection of sinew to bone, we can use acupressure rather than puncturing techniques.

LU-10 has a similar function to LU-3 in that it can be used to treat sadness and fear. This point has the added benefit of addressing dysfunction such as esophageal spasm and blood in the urine. The first is fairly common when a patient has a weak neck. Blood in urine requires biomedical intervention. However, LU-10 can be used to ameliorate discomfort while the patient is in the process of working with their MD to identify causes and establish a safe protocol for resolution. This is also a good point for trigger thumb, though of course we would take care with weak tissue, no matter how contracted and dense it might seem.

Returning to the source, we remember that the Lung channel originates in the middle Jiao at the region of the Stomach and that the channel's meeting place with the Spleen is at its first point, LU-1. Zhongfu, or Middle Palace, is the front Mu point of the Lung and can be used for respiratory difficulty or for skin pain. It is close enough to the shoulder joint that one must take care. Patients with very stretchy skin, especially, are not good candidates for acupuncture here or at LU-2. Gentle tui na, which I discuss in chapter five, is better. In my experience, the declaration that zhongfu is, "[...] one of the few acupuncture points indicated for the painful skin which can consequently accompany exterior diseases" (Deadman *et al.* 2007, p.77) also holds true for hEDS. But carefully, carefully, especially if the patient has an unstable shoulder. Nurturing the qi of LU-1 and SP-21 in a treatment can ameliorate a number of manifestations of pain, both internal and on the skin, that one might expect to see in an hEDS patient.

One might produce volumes regarding the taiyin channel of the foot and its organ, the Spleen. This is a central organ and substantive channel for all patients, but for a patient with hEDS?

The plight of the malfunctioning Spleen is writ large on the body of a person who is built with malfunctioning connective tissue.

When there is easy bruising, as is common, we can identify the Spleen not controlling the Blood. People with hEDS often have icy cold feet and hands; again, a tangible demonstration of the Spleen's malfunction. The Spleen controls the muscles and flesh. A patient who presents with muscle atrophy and soft, stretchy flesh is an example of the Spleen in the context of qi and yang deficiency. The Spleen regulates the upbearing of qi in the digestive process. Accessing nutrition from the food as it undergoes the digestive process also falls under the purview of the Spleen. When we speak of gastroparesis and inability to take in and process nutrition, either from the perspective of calories or macro and micro nutrients, this is the Spleen's responsibility. When our patients experience organ prolapse or ptosis, that is Spleen qi sinking. When their Blood fails to warm and nourish them, again, it is the Spleen.

The Spleen also pertains to worry. In the case of hEDS, the patient may be a textbook example of the relationship of Spleen to overthinking. They may suffer from chronic, low-grade (or extreme, depending) anxiety, and they may have a propensity for intrusive thoughts and endless looping rumination. Living in a body in pain can exacerbate unrelenting disquiet. On a subconscious level, I am convinced that the body knows, after its own fashion, that bones are in danger of slipping out of place at any given moment. This puts the body on a chronic hum of low-grade anxiety that never quite goes away. That, in an hEDS patient, is the Spleen stepping up to its appointed task of ruminating and worry.

The Spleen is the mantle that covers all hEDS concerns. It is the center of all issues. A practitioner will center the Spleen when treating an hEDS patient whether or not we are a follower of the Earth School of Chinese medicine. The Spleen is the center of all matter herein.

The points that we select to treat the above-mentioned conditions are the same as the ones we would use for a patient who does not live with HCTD. Certain points (SP-6, 9, and 10, for instance) are excellent when they are indicated, and they are excellent for all patients, not just our hEDS ones. What do require particular attention in the instance of hEDS are specific considerations relating to tensile strength of the tissue itself, location, and comparative values.

SP-9, or yinlingquan (Yin Mound Spring), is a useful clue for connective tissue disorder. A person with hEDS may have a soft, puffy area at this point that differs from what we palpate on someone with Dampness issues but not an HCTD. A patient with a soft, puffy SP-9 point may also have a gummy nodule on ST-40. On these patients, the Spleen point will feel as though there is uncooked biscuit dough under a piece of silk and the puffy subsurface will be relatively warm. On other patients, the feeling is more as though there is a divot. It feels like the practitioner could press and their fingers would come out on the other side of the knee, at ST-36. These patients, for their part, will have a spot that feels like a Phlegm nodule on SP-10 or at ST-36. Palpating SP-9 with sensitive fingers and being ready to check either ST-36 or 40 or SP-10 in response to the relative texture can be informative.

Learning to distinguish between the tissue of a person with an HCTD as compared with someone without can occur just by paying attention to SP-9. The same potential for discovery is in SP-10 as well, but not to the degree one finds with Yin Mound Spring.

Of all the points on the Spleen, the end-point, SP-21, is fascinating. I remember learning about it in one or the other of my first-year courses and thinking, "Oh, yes, I know this point!" When I was in my first graduate program and studying for my Ph.D. qualifying exams (twenty grueling hours of three six-hour written exams and one two-hour oral defense), my SP-21 point would spontaneously gush perspiration, as though it had turned into a little water spout. This was well before I had ever heard of

Chinese medicine, to be clear. And yes, I experienced this as my program in Chinese medicine progressed. It happens only when there is a confluence of extreme fatigue and high-level anxiety, but my left-side SP-21 apparently turns into a waterfall when exams loom and I feel threatened and am exhausted. When treating hEDS patients, I have found that tui na can produce spontaneous sweating on one or both SP-21 points when the patient is very tired or extremely anxious. Bringing this perspiration to the surface seems to be a release and quite relaxing for the patient.

All quirks related to perspiration aside, we will recollect that this is a Luo point known as dabao (Great Wrapping). According to the Spiritual Pivot, "When it is excess, there is pain of the whole body. When it is deficient the hundred joints are flaccid. This channel embraces the blood of all the luo" (quoted in *ibid.*, p.204). A practitioner who works with hEDS patients will learn to read this point with the same dedication that is shown to SP-9, and to treat it with great respect for its healing properties. If I had to choose only three Spleen points and never use another, I would take SP-6, 9, and 21 for my hypermobile patients. I learn from what they tell me and they, in turn, serve the patient well when I correctly manipulate the flow of qi therein.

## Shaoyin Channel and Organs

Reading reports of fieldwork in China undertaken by anthropologists can, at times, unearth clinical pearls. Sometimes, they will leave a reader saddened. "Once I was amused by a patient," writes Yanhua Zhang, "who complained that he could feel his heartbeat everywhere on his body, and he insisted that wherever on his body he touched, he could count his heartbeat" (2007, p.78). The narrative does not make it clear why this would be amusing, but she is an anthropologist and I am a clinician so of course our interpretations may differ. Indeed, experience with HCTD patients shifts perspectives about such matters as palpitations that are extremely real to the patient but potentially not decipherable via Chinese or Western medicine. It is not rare to treat hEDS patients who have tachycardia, either because they have POTS or because they can feel every beat of their heart due to causes unknown. This patient may have had FMD, POTS, or an HCTD. Perhaps he was neurodivergent and able to feel his own body in a way that a less-sensitive person could not.

Fortunately, the physician of record did not find the man's suffering risible. Zhang relates that, "Afterward, the doctor seriously said to me that we healthy people may never experience what the patient experiences, but that doesn't mean that what the patient experiences isn't real or relevant" (*ibid.*, p.78).

My experience is such that several of my patients have reported being unable to relax at night due to a sense that they can hear their heart pounding in their chest or feel it up in their ears when they are in bed and trying to sleep. If I had a patient tell me that they could feel their heartbeat everywhere in their body, I would believe them and think it unsurprising, especially if I palpated their Heart channel and determined that they were hypermobile or in some way spongier than a person with "normal" connective tissue would be. Individuals with hEDS often have palpitations that are unique to their presentations. Most times, their MD can determine why this is so; other times, nobody knows. Either way, the patient's experience is real.

As Deadman *et al.* remind, palpitations are considered in three categories. These are: relatively unremarkable palpitations, those accompanied or triggered by the sensation of fear, and "pounding of the Heart (the most serious kind) which denotes palpitations that can be felt as high up as the heart itself or as low as the umbilicus (the termination point of the Heart sinew channel)" (2007, p.227). HT-5 is particularly relevant in this instance, as is HT-7. We might also take note of any signs of Wind, especially if this is a patient with MCAS or dysautonomia plus urticaria. Patients who have idiopathic palpitations and who have been cleared by their MD for any organ malfunction will sometimes respond very well to herbal treatment designed to mitigate the effects of Wind. In addition, one might try, in these cases, specific Wind points like GB-20, DU-24, or the Extra point baichongwo if we opt for a Gu syndrome as our starting point.

The Heart as an organ governs the Blood and Blood vessels and has an intimate relationship with the Lungs, its canopy. Together, these organs control the gathering qi (zong qi) that regulates breath and circulation of blood. The Heart also regulates sweating. This organ opens into the tongue, houses the shen, and expresses itself in the facial complexion. In the context of hEDS, the Heart is particularly worthy of focus when it comes to shen disturbance, difficulty regulating the autonomic nervous system, and the aforementioned palpitations. The Heart in its interior/exterior relationship with the Small Intestine is relevant when treating patients who suffer from repeated UTIs. It is also worth considering the Heart if the patient experiences ocular disorders.

As a student intern, I had a patient who suffered from air hunger. In this instance, the Heart channel was telling. This patient had undergone endless diagnostic tests, and no useful determination was made. This patient simply had to live with the constant sense of not having enough air. And, while her blood oxygen values did fluctuate, they did not do so to the degree that the patient's discomfort suggested. Her doctors eventually recommended that she try acupuncture. At the time, I had only been studying hEDS for a couple of years and I did not have enough experience to ask good questions. What I did find on palpation, though, were soft areas of the medial arm that were punctuated by gummy nodules. I decided to focus on LU-5 and HT-3 and thread needles towards each other on either arm. Among other points now lost to my memory, I recollect that I added LU-3 and PC-6 plus yintang and KD-3 to the prescription.

When the joints are unstable, the fascia gets tugged here and there, and the qi circulation becomes disrupted. The patient was unable to relax and take a deep breath, but by releasing blockages and nourishing qi circulation, she was able to experience respite. Even now, I remember this patient because seeing her face become peaceful touched me so. Like most student interns, I was unsure of myself in the clinical space, and this felt like such a success! For a time, she could nap and feel able to breathe. I do not know if this was a patient with an HCTD but if someone came to me today with her presentation, I would palpate the Heart and Lung channels in search of answers and I would look for clues suggestive of dysautonomia. I might also identify a syndrome pattern of Kidney not grasping the qi, compounded by Lungs weakened by grief, and deficiency of Heart Blood.

Another issue that plagues an hEDS body is prolapse. Though we will categorize this as a matter of Spleen qi sinking, it can be useful to recollect that the bao mai pertains to the Heart and is connected with the uterus. A treatment that configures Heart involvement might also rely on the point HT-8 when addressing uterine prolapse.

When working with HCTDs, our approach to the Kidney organs and channel is not going to be radically different than it be would when treating any other patient. As an umbrella category, both organ and channel hold the same significance for patients regardless of the state of their connective tissue. In other words: either it is relevant to the patient's ailment or it is not. There is no need for an hEDS-specific lens with which to view the Kidney or the foot shaoyin channel. The Kidney organ is not necessarily exceptional when treating patients with HCTD. The way we might nourish Kidney yang for treatment of erectile dysfunction in a patient without hEDS is not going to be too different than the way we would treat these syndromes in someone with hEDS. And yet, certain characteristics of hEDS in the Kidney, both organ and channel, hold certain points of interest for the specialist.

We will keep in mind that, "Its original yin provides the material foundation for human development and reproduction, and its original yang promotes and activates the vital functions of the bowels and viscera" (Yán and Lǐ 2012, p.1). The Kidneys pertain to the process of storing essence and fostering reproduction, growth, and development. The Kidneys house the vital essence, and our treatment strategies will focus on nourishing jing of patients with or in the absence of hEDS. They open into the ears and regulate the two lower yin (anus and urethra). The Kidneys house the will. The basis of our medical ideology is founded on the interrelatedness of all processes. We keep in mind that, "the Kidneys occupy a unique position among the *zangfu*, both storing the yin essence and conserving and controlling the ming men fire. The Kidneys are thus the root of the yin and yang of the whole body. Because of this fundamental role, deficiency of the Kidneys may both cause and result from disharmony of any of the other *zangfu*" (Deadman *et al.* 2007, p.340).

Dr. Wang reminds that, "The shao yin organs are also responsible for maintaining the body's warmth. This is different from the spleen taiyin function of warming the yin organs. Taiyin warming is provided by nourishment while shao yin warming is provided by the movement of blood and the physiological fundamentals of the gate of vitality and sovereign fire" (Wang and Robertson 2008, p.102). With respect to Heat and Fire in the channels, Dr. Wang notes that this could be excess or it may be deficiency. "However," he explains, "—and this is important—if the ultimate cause is related to shao yin, then there is deficiency at the root. In other words, while channel symptoms may often look like excess, the underlying dysfunction in shao yin is deficiency" (*ibid.*, p.103). People with hEDS tend towards Cold and deficiency. The observation that, "Damp fluids can lead to cold; thus long, clear, profuse urination is a sign that the body is trying to remove fluids in an effort to create net warmth. This type of urination, in fact, is often a symptom of cold from deficiency in the kidneys" (*ibid.*, p.111) is noteworthy for patients who experience nocturia that fits Dr. Wang's description. Points that can be useful here are KD-3 and 15.

Because uterine prolapse is a concern for this demographic, we keep in mind specific points that we might employ in its treatment. We might opt to include KD-5 or 8 in our point prescription, noting that KD-8 is at the joint. Depending on the texture and relative strength of the tendons, it is wise to needle gently or avoid KD-8 when treating fragile patients. KD-3 is an excellent point, of course. It is a point used to tonify the yang, anchor qi, and benefit the Lung, and it strengthens the lumbar spine. Like points at the knee joint, it is wise to consider tensile strength of the ankles before placing needles at KD-3. KD-26 is useful for treating pityriasis versicolor, though I am more inclined to use ear seeds to stimulate this point given its location.

A useful point for navicular syndrome is KD-2. Interestingly, I have treated hEDS patients with one foot that is cold and the other that is relatively warm, and, of course, anything that we can do to address pain is always helpful. Deadman *et al.*'s list of indications for this point is relevant, "One foot hot and one foot cold, pain of the lower legs which prevents standing for long periods, pain and swelling of the instep..." (2007, p.338). Combining this point with SP-7 and 8 can provide pain relief for patients with Bi syndrome.

## Jueyin Channel and Organs

The Pericardium organ's name sums up its function as an entity. The xin bao, or Heart's Wrapper, protects the Heart from exterior pathogens. As one of my Chinese teachers would say, "The Heart is the emperor and thus lazy. He lets the Pericardium do all the work." This organ does not have its own Shu points and it is discussed in classical literature solely as the protector of the Heart. The channel, for its part, is useful for treating disorders of the Heart organ and, given that palpitations can be an issue with hEDS, it is worth keeping this in mind for the treatment of same. The channel is noteworthy for treating local pain and upper body pain due to Liver qi stagnation. It is good for treating the psyche as well.

The more useful points start at PC-3, and discussion of this point is a perfect opportunity to remind practitioners that joints in an hEDS body can be *somewhat* unstable or they can be *incredibly* unstable. A patient with a wobbly neck or cervical pain will probably have fragile forearms. Palpation may reveal a crispy feel to the subsurface of the skin, or the practitioner will notice remarkably loose or tight joints at elbow and/or wrist. Arms like this respond better to ear seeds than they do to acupuncture needles. PC-3 is good for Heart pain and disordered rhythm and, as I mentioned regarding a patient I saw as an intern, it can be useful for air hunger. Using seeds on HT-3 and PC-3 together can be most efficacious indeed. Adding BL-40 to this combination, especially with seeds, can be useful for patients who struggle to maintain a calm Heart spirit and relaxed limbs.

Generally, an hEDS patient will not present with Heat symptoms. It is more common to see patients who suffer from freezing hands and feet. Consequently PC-4's value in treating Heat in the Blood that disturbs the Heart is not common. However, the connection between Heart qi and Blood makes this a point to use for insomnia, anxiety, and fearfulness. PC-5, just down the line towards the wrist, is a valuable tool for treating palpitations and, like ST-40, it is a point used to treat disorders involving Phlegm. This point also regulates the Stomach via its internal/external connection with the San Jiao channel and is especially valuable when treating patients with dysautonomia. PC-5 can also be used in cases of prolapsed rectum.

PC-6 is of course excellent for nausea, as is PC-9, though we will recollect that a patient with intractable nausea may be suffering from MALS.

PC-7 is a valuable point for palpitations, extremes of emotion, and contraction of the hand. Given that hEDS patients tend to suffer from trigger finger or thumb, this is a useful point to keep in mind. However, it is important to remember that it's on the joint, and it is wise to be gentle with it. PC-8 is helpful in cases of hemorrhoids and/or painful hand obstruction, although in my experience, tui na on these points can be just as, if not more, effective while needles here can be painful. These are points that elicit a strong reaction and it is smart to be mindful and rely on warming techniques rather than aggressive stimulation.

From hand to foot, the jueyin channel is significant in the treatment of HCTD patients, and the organs are no less so. The Liver organ and the Spleen are foundational organs for addressing hEDS. While the Spleen pertains to the muscles, the Liver regulates the sinews. We all know that the Liver stores blood and maintains the free flow of qi, and keep in mind that the Liver opens into the eyes and manifests in the fingernails. The normal state of affairs is that the Liver overacts on the Spleen but, interestingly enough, with hEDS a practitioner might find that the Liver pulse seems worn and flaccid while the Spleen pulse is energetic, as if the Spleen were overacting on the Liver.

The distal points of the Liver channel are good for treating urinary disorders. In instances of ptosis, an hEDS patient can be treated using LV-1 or 2 in combination with SP-6 and other prolapse points like DU-20. LV-1 can be used to address blood in the urine. LV-3 and the classic combination that is Four Gates can be relied upon to treat hEDS patients the way that they can with any other patients, albeit with a caveat. To wit: patients with evident Wind conditions (hives, urticaria) react strongly to the LI-4 point. More than once, I had patients who developed a rash from the metacarpal joint of the index finger to its tip at LI-1, and I eventually learned to avoid using Four Gates on patients with MCAS if they were either in a flare or coming out of one. I will always use LV-3 when the patient has trigger finger or other contraction of the hand.

LV-6 is useful for patients who roll their ankles or who have weak, painful feet. Being positioned midway on the lower limb, rather than at a joint, makes LV-6 a good point for both clinical efficacy and patient safety.

LV-4 and 6 are good for treating men's problems. Erectile dysfunction is distressing for any guy, but as part of the hEDS presentation, it is challenging because the matter may not only be low testosterone but, instead, can include the outcome of having weak connective tissue throughout the body. It can be useful to set aside the question of yang qi at first, and focus more on nourishing the channel. Concurrently, we treat for Spleen qi sinking (i.e., prolapse) and Cold. In such patients, we may also note Dampness. Palpation and visual inspection may reveal a puffy, soft bed of flesh covering the lower back and lumbo-sacral junction. One might also see distended or blue-green veins across the sacrum. Resolving the Dampness and overabundance of yin first can make addressing Kidney yang qi easier subsequently.

LV-8 is helpful in the instance of erectile dysfunction but, given that it is at the knee joint and close to tendons, it does require mindful application. It is also useful for uterine prolapse, with the same caveat. LV-13 harmonizes the Liver and Spleen, "when qi stagnation aggressively invades, obstructs and suppresses the transportation and transformation function of the Spleen, or from the Spleen, when Spleen qi deficiency is unable to resist the encroachment of exuberant Liver qi" (Deadman *et al.* 2007, p.489). In the case of hEDS, it usually a matter of Spleen qi deficiency unable to defend itself against the Liver; either way, I tend to put ear seeds on these points rather than needles, especially if the patient is one who has weak ribs.

## Taiyang Channel and Organs

The Small Intestine, Heart's pair, is a Fire channel and its connections with the Bladder channel and pathways make it uniquely relevant to the clearing of Heat. This is not always useful in the case of hEDS, given that this is a population that tends towards Cold. In addition, though the Small Intestine is tasked with receiving, transporting, and separating fluids, this organ is not generally used for treating digestive difficulties. Comparatively, we will note that, per classical thought, "While the large intestine is compared to a pathway, the small intestine is viewed as a brief stopping point for assimilation and modification"; concurrently, "the stomach is likened to an official charged with the collection of grains, and the small intestine to a lower functionary charged with classification" (Wang and Robertson 2008, pp.189–190).

Small Intestine points treat pain. As Deadman *et al.* observe, SI-3 is an essential point for treating occipital headache and neck stiffness, and this point, "has a significant effect on the spine as a whole" (2007, p.234). SI-4, for its part, is worth using for muscle contracture along the channel itself. We note, as well, that SI-7 is helpful for, "slackness of the joints and inability to move the elbow" (*ibid.*, p.239), though my experience when using this point for hEDS treatment is that either tui na or ear seeds are gentle and efficacious approaches while needling tends to overstimulate the channel. SI-18 and 19 particularly, especially for patients who suffer from jaw pain and/or dental issues, are valuable in one's treatment strategy. According to Dr. Liu, "All tetany and stiff neck belongs to dampness," and he asserts that, "Nowadays, we see a lot of cervical spine disorders. All of this cervical pathology can be considered and treated from the perspective of Taiyang and Taiyin" (2019, p.260).

The Small Intestine channel is a diagnostic tool. According to Dr. Wang, neck and shoulder ligament dysfunction can be reflected on the SI channel and, if so, a practitioner might look to the line between SI-3 and 6 for nodules; further, he notes, "Sometimes back pain manifesting on the bladder tài yang channel will manifest on the small intestine channel" and in such cases, the practitioner may look to the contralateral SI-3 point for confirmation (Wang and Robertson 2008, p.192). SI-9 and 10, commonly used to treat shoulder pain, are tremendously helpful in response to aches associated with hEDS and tight shoulders. Points closer to the midline and spine require special care in patients whose soft tissue is silky and thin. Needles can go in deeper and faster than one might expect when treating an hEDS patient. I personally tend to avoid points on the neck (SI-16 and 17) for this reason.

The Bladder is a yang organ, tasked with removing waste from the body in the form of urine. Paired with the Kidneys, the Bladder's element is Water. As an organ, its greatest claim to fame (or at least reason for interest) is that it pairs with the Kidney; meanwhile, in practice, we tend to focus on the channel more than the organ. When treating patients with hEDS, the Bladder organ becomes a focus because bladder pain is common in this population. A practitioner who sees HCTD patients will eventually become well versed in bladder dysfunction from both Eastern and Western perspectives. This can be due to Spleen qi sinking. It can be the result of chronic low-level inflammation caused by hypersensitivity or MCAS, thereby falling under categories like Heat or Wind. A pelvic floor plagued with Blood stasis and Cold might also be a factor.

How much we make use of the full range of points can vary. Perhaps, we simply rely on the back Shu points, the front Mu, a couple of the initial points, and a handful of distal points. In *Applied Channel Theory*, Dr. Wang's thoughts in this regard are instructive. He reminds us that, "the key to consistent use of any concept in Chinese medicine depends on a clear understanding in the doctor's mind of the diagnosis. The clearer the diagnosis, the more precise the treatment" (*ibid.*, p.206). In choosing points, he says that each has its own nature and talents, just as people do. According to Dr. Wang:

> Some people are adept at doing a wide variety of things: jacks-of-all-trades. Other people have only very specific skills. Commonly used acupuncture points like ST-36, SP-6, CV-12, and GB-34 are points of very broad application. On the other hand, other points that are rarely used have very precise applications for particular illnesses. In the case of these rarely used points, the key is to get to know them. One must know their specific strengths and not attempt to apply them too broadly. This, to me, is one of the most subtle and difficult aspects of acupuncture to teach. Experience and careful study is the only way to get to know the very precise personalities of some of the points. (*ibid.*, p.206)

The context of this wise teacher's remarks pertains to Bladder points on the back. However, when working with HCTDs, we develop our capacity by considering and reconsidering the points and their value to hEDS bodies. Different points do have different personalities in such cases, and each practitioner will bring their gifts to the table in unique ways. Some of us are able to achieve great success for our patients via the broad application. Others of us will specialize and rely on rarely used points. Precision in diagnosis and careful study remain our watchwords, and as we become experienced, we develop our reliance on one point rather than another.[8]

BL-2, at the medial aspect of the eyebrows directly above the inner canthus of the eye, and BL-3, just above it and a half cun into the hairline, offer a useful example. The points are good for Wind, headache, eye pain, and rhinitis. Because they are not on joints, they are usually well tolerated, even by the most flexible of hEDS patient, but keep in mind that BL-2 is not a good idea for patients who bruise easily. In the instance of cEDS, which is characterized by extremely silky and loose skin, we might avoid BL-2 in favor of BL-3 only (and needle upward, towards the top of the scalp), but these are safe and effective points for most patients. Moving upward and across the scalp to BL-9, it is possible to treat allergy or MCAS without worry. With BL-10, as with GB-20, we take great care with patients who have hyperflexible necks. Practice and familiarity with a range of EDS presentations will make needling Bladder points up and over the scalp easier and easier.

The back Shu points that we routinely use with great success hold true for HCTD patients. What needs to be factored in is the relative softness of the tissue and the condition of the ribs and their connection to the spine. In the instance of Bladder points on the back, the first determining factor is not that this or the other is a good point for this or that syndrome. Instead, it is an issue of whether or not the person's body is capable of being safely needled. In addition, these are points that can be extremely reactive when a patient has MCAS or any form of dysautonomia. We start with a needle or two and see what happens before overdoing it on the Bladder lines of the back. This holds especially true for the outer Bladder line and even more so if the patient is thin.

Moving down the back of the leg, it is most important to factor in stability of joints. As lovely a point as BL-40 is, we need to be attentive to how strong the knee is before needling this one and its neighbors, BL-38 and 39. BL-57, so good for hemorrhoids, is usually a safe and easy point to needle. Moving down to the ankle requires focus so as not to disrupt uneasy attachment of tendon to bone. BL-60 and 61 are wonderful points for the frequent headaches common to hEDS but the practitioner will wish to have a good sense of whether or not the person's foot is unstable before making use of them.

## Shaoyang Channel and Organs

Interiorly/exteriorly coupled with the Pericardium channel and paired with the Gall Bladder channel of the foot shaoyang, the

San Jiao is another channel that specifically is used to address Heat. Though not precisely an organ, the San Jiao is relevant to HCTD in that this entity encompasses a concept akin to that of the interstitium.[9] It is divided into three, with the first being the upper Jiao, which pertains to the Heart and the Lung and supports breathing and air metabolism. The middle Jiao, which constitutes the digestive system and its processes, holds within its purview the separation of the pure and impure, a process that begins in the upper realms of this sector. Subsequently, the impure passes to the lower Jiao for elimination. Its layers can be conceptualized as mist (upper), foam (middle), and swamp (lower).

In the context of hEDS, the San Jiao as a concept is relevant. When we consider that metabolism is often disrupted, it can be helpful to distance one's view enough to see things from the upper/middle/lower perspective and through the lens of metabolism. Conversely, if we do view the San Jiao as the original interstitium, this makes sense in its capacity a visceral organ. Whichever way that we choose to interpret this concept, it is helpful to keep in mind that, as Dr. Wang asserts in *Applied Channel Theory*, "The concept of the triple burner is one of the most debated topics of historical Chinese medical literature" (Wang and Robertson 2008, p.216). And yet, as he explains, "All of the myriad transformations of qi, at every moment during the process of metabolism, are occurring within the environments maintained by the triple burner"; consequently, if we locate this within Western terms, we keep in mind that, "in modern physiological terms, the triple burner might be thought to represent the fluid pathways within which the complex process of cellular metabolism occurs" (*ibid.*, p.217).[10]

Absent a precise definition of the San Jiao as an organ, we will be confident treating patients via direct engagement with the specific points and the overall channel.

Treating via the fingers in hEDS can be safer than needling

larger joints. For this reason, SJ-1 is useful for addressing earache (so common with hEDS, due to TMJ disorder). SJ-2 is useful for local symptoms of pain and contracture in the hand and wrist in addition to calming the spirit. We take care with this one, as some patients have exceptionally hypermobile fingers and wrists. SJ-3 is good for ear pain but SJ-4, unless the patient has sturdy wrists, is best avoided. SJ-5 is a gem of a point for issues that plague anyone with an HCTD, including: headache, ear pain, eye pain, stiffness of the tongue, toothache, and stiffness of the elbow and arm. We remember to be careful here, though. I have had patients who could not handle even the finest needle in their SJ-5, but with ear seeds, they felt an incredible sense of pain relief. We choose wisely where we needle on the forearm with some patients. SJ-6 is good for all of the above plus it can be helpful in cases of constipation. Our gastroparesis patients will thank us for judicious use of SJ-6.

SJ-7, 8, 9, and 10 are also useful for pain, ear problems, and toothache. When we get to SJ-10, it is best to skip unless actively treating for Heat and Phlegm disorders. This is an area best suited to gentle tui na or maybe cupping with delicate cups normally used for facial rejuvenation. The upper reaches of the San Jiao on the arm continue in this theme; essentially, though, the ones at the joint are tricky for unstable connections and best left to either gentle manual therapies or the thermal design power (TDP) lamp plus ear seeds. SJ-17 is absolutely and without question an excellent point for unstable, painful necks, but it takes a careful hand to place the needle and trust between practitioner and patient. Having Eagle syndrome, especially in cases of vEDS, can make this point dangerous for the patient.[11]

The points that surround the ear, starting with SJ-17 and continuing through to SJ-22, are invaluable for ear and tooth pain. Tinnitus and headache also respond well to these points. SJ-23, especially if used along with yuyao and BL-2, are helpful for sinus issues, eye pain, head Wind, and other similar. Caveat:

as we know, people with hEDS can bruise spectacularly and easy-bruising patient will not thank us for marking their forehead and brows with purple.

The Gall Bladder's two main functions are to store and excrete bile and, on an intangible level, this organ pertains to courage and decision-making. From the perspective of the channel and points, the Gall Bladder is most useful for treating Wind, Heat, and/or Phlegm. Certain points are especially useful for responding to eye and ear problems. Gall Bladder points can be used to clear pathogen at the shaoyang level, to treat disorders of the Liver, and to ameliorate certain types of muscle pain and atrophy.

As ever, there are points that are specifically useful for hEDS patients and some will have their caveats. GB-2, for instance, is a tremendously useful point for treating TMJ disorder and Bell's palsy but, given its location, it requires extra attention. If the patient has a history of jaw dislocation, this is cause for consideration. If, on the other hand, the patient has a painfully tight jaw that spasms, looking ahead to the outcome of loosening it is the concern. What might happen if the TMJ is released? In a non-hEDS patient, this would probably result in pain relief and joy. With hEDS, it might mean that a tight jaw is now one that boomerangs to its opposite condition and dislocates.[12] Before working directly on the local area, it can be helpful to experiment and see how the patient responds to distal treatment first. It is always good to try things out on a less-fraught region and see what happens before working directly on a joint.

GB-8 is a potent point for Wind, nausea, and pain. Interestingly, my clinical experience has been such that this point is exceptionally useful for rashes of unknown origin. I have found that it works especially well for people with MCAS.[13]

GB-12 and 13 (the latter especially when used with DU-24) are useful for brain fog, poor memory, and local problems like headache and neck stiffness. It is useful to take note of relative laxity of the cervical spine before treating via this area, but both GB-12 and 20 seem, for most, to not result in untoward outcomes. That's not the case for all hEDS patients. I've had some whose sub-occipitals are strictly the purview of their osteopath or chiropractor. But in general, these are good points. GB-14 is a wonderful point for trigeminal neuralgia, and the patient can be taught to self-massage the forehead gently for home care. GB-15 is useful for sinusitis and other problems related to the nose and eyes. Any of the points on the scalp can usually be employed without consideration for the muscles and fascia (though of course we would take note of any undue Wind-related reactions). Especially with thin patients, I only use ear seeds on GB-21.

GB-34, or Yang Mound Spring, is one of the most important points we can use when treating patients with HCTDs. This is the magic point for just about any hEDS patient, and how it factors into the overall treatment plan depends on whichever other points the practitioner will want to use. It is exceptional for pain, stiffness, and contraction of the sinews. As we will learn from the *Song of Points for Miscellaneous Diseases*, this point is excellent for pain of the lateral costal region; further, the *Ode of Essentials of Understanding* avers that, "when there is pain of the lateral costal region and the ribs, needling Yanglingquan GB-34 will alleviate the pain promptly" (quoted in Deadman *et al.* 2007, p.451). In my experience, this is a useful point for costal pain. For patients with HCTDs, GB-34 is the equivalent of ST-36. It's the magic point. I have never felt concerned about needling GB-34 with any of my patients, and if I had only one Gall Bladder point to use, it would have to be this one (unless the patient had MCAS, and then I would need to go with GB-8).

People with hEDS often have painful feet, and treating systemic issues via foot points can be an excellent strategy. GB-41 is best accessed with tui na, as needles can be overly stimulating for a patient who has flat feet or otherwise deals with chronic foot problems. It is generally safe to needle GB-43 without undue concern, and GB-44 remains useful for the treatment of nightmares, somnolence, and other sleep disorders. It is also good for contracted sinews.

## Yangming Channel and Organs

We are all familiar with what Chapter 9 of the *Spiritual Pivot* has to say about this area, "Yangming channel is abundant in qi and blood" (quoted in Deadman *et al.* 2007, p.129). Thus we are well aware of the value of relying on this channel to treat pain and weakness. The organs are relevant to an HCTD presentation in ways similar to any other patient and, for the most part, the points one will choose are more or less the same in either instance. More or less. As with everything else, there are at least a few details that relate to working with HCTD patients.

The Large Intestine sinew channel, rather than the primary meridian, is often the most painful for hEDS patients. When we might turn to the Large Intestine channel of the hand, we eventually focus instead on the sinew channel because we will see, in patient after patient, that this is where things hurt the most. As a concept, we will recollect that the Lung's paired organ is tasked with the less-glamorous job of extracting nutrients and compacting the detritus before expelling it as waste. In this way, the Large Intestine organ is an intrinsic aspect of the digestive process and thus within the axis of the Spleen/Stomach's duties. When the Large Intestine is a focus of the treatment strategy, it is, on a broad level, either due to its psycho-emotional role of letting go (or not) or because there is a Large Intestine sinew channel issue, in which case we are dealing with pain. For hEDS patients, we will very often rely on channel theory and the Large Intestine channel to resolve or ameliorate said pain.

A patient whose body is constantly "letting go" might react by hanging on in other areas, and in this case, we might consider referencing the Large Intestine. Grief and sorrow are the Lung's emotions and can be expressed (or not) via the yin organ's yang pair. It can be worthwhile to palpate the forearm with an eye for the metaphysical in such cases.

It is worth mentioning again that I do not needle LI-4 when a patient is experiencing or recovering from an MCAS flare-up. As per Deadman *et al.*, LI-4, "regulates the defensive qi and adjusts sweating" and, "expels wind and releases the exterior" (2007, p.103). What that can mean for a person with MCAS, at least in my experience, is a startling red rash that goes all the way to the finger's edge at LI-1. Interestingly, LI-20, on the other end, does not cause such a reaction and I will use it with MCAS patients. Not LI-4 though.

The Stomach is responsible for down-bearing energy and matter. In concert with the Spleen, the Stomach is responsible for the digestive system and its functions. Poor appetite and failure to thrive are traced back to these organs. We do keep in mind that nausea might not just be Stomach qi rebellion. As mentioned, there are particular considerations with hEDS patients, one of which is the weakness of Spleen qi allowing the flesh to easily move and the vessels to become pressed.

The same points that we rely on with our non-HCTD patients will work just as well for our people with hEDS. We consider location and tensile strength before placing needles, just as we do with every other point. What can be unique to the Stomach channel and points, in any event, is that same notion of *and what else?* that I mentioned in chapter two regarding digestive health. Does the patient experience bloating and hives when they eat? It might be that the patient is constipated and they experience angioedema under their eyes or on their lips in response to food. Someone else might consume nothing but be fat, while the next person eats and eats but cannot maintain their weight. There is almost always this *and what else?* factor when we focus on the yangming organs, especially with respect to the Stomach.

This channel and its organs are famous for being abundant

in qi and Blood so we remember to expand our perspective to include the full syndrome pattern surrounding not just it but also the ripples in the pond created by whatever stones are dropped therein.[14]

## The Ren and the Du Vessels and Points

As an extraordinary vessel, the Ren is the yin to the Du's yang. To speak of one side is to acknowledge the other, for they are a pair. Li Shi-zhen notes that:

> The Conception and Governing vessels are like midnight and midday, they are the polar axis of the body...there is one source and two branches, one goes to the front and the other to the back of the body... When we try to divide these, we see that yin and yang are inseparable. When we try to see them as one, we see an indivisible whole. (quoted in Deadman *et al.* 2007, p.496)

When we include points from these channels, we can rely on them in many of the same ways that we would for any patient. However, there are, of course, some particular considerations to keep in mind when needling or otherwise stimulating the points on the Du and the Ren vessels.

How we choose one point or another based on anatomy and relative safety for an unstable body is always our first concern. It is a good idea to avoid Du points on the neck, for instance. I am disinclined to needle any Du point on the spine but ear seeds can be optimal in this area. I do like points on the scalp because they tend to be safe for unstable bodies, and the points in question are useful. Needling HT-8, PC-6, and threading DU-23 to DU-24 can an excellent base formula when a patient has nightmares, for example, and I may be inclined to put ear seeds on KD-1 in such cases as well. The scalp points are like having a twenty-dollar bill in your back pocket that can be used in case of unexpected need. They are nice to have around.

Tui na on DU-15 and 16 after surgery for Chiari can be soothing and healing if we are gentle and kind with our hands. DU-26 is good for Bell's palsy and trigeminal neuralgia, both of which we will not be surprised to see in our hEDS patients.

Because people with hEDS are more vulnerable to pelvic organ prolapse we will find ourselves relying on both DU and REN-4 more than we might otherwise. We might be able to help stave off surgery with herbal medicine and judicious acupuncture treatment on the lower abdomen. After the patient has had surgery, if things have come to that, we can support their healing process with Du and Ren points on the lower abdomen and sacral area. Personally, I would not be inclined to treat a patient with either DU or REN-1. It is more prudent to let the urogynecologist refer our patient to a PT who specializes in pelvic floor health.

The Ren points on the abdomen are useful and oft-employed points for patients with digestive difficulty. However, we remain mindful of the patient's body. Their abdomen may be covered with cigarette-paper scars or silky stretch marks and visible blue veins. These patients might have a better reaction to either very fine, small needles or ear seeds. My experience with lower backs that seem spongy and laced with remarkable veins is that acupuncture improves the tissue strength but it takes time and consistency. I like REN-24 a lot for Bell's palsy, although it is important to support a weak neck before needling into this point. The small wrist pillows used for pulse diagnosis make excellent neck pillows for hEDS patients in such instances.

## The Extraordinary Points

The Extraordinary points follow the pattern we have seen thus far. In other words: where is the point and is it one that addresses specific issues that we will often see with hEDS? Sishencong is a useful set of points and not one to cause issues with lax patients. Since this requires four needles, it might be overly stimulating for a person with dysautonomia, and we might in that case rely on DU-20 instead. Yintang might not always be the best due to bleeding or bruising. Ear points tend to be safe, and erjian is no different. Anmian is great as long as the patient doesn't have an overly loose neck. Jiachengjiang is useful for local problems of the shoulder, although I avoid that one for patients with unstable shoulder joints. Zigong and tituo are important points for prolapse, and we will use them regularly unless the patient is extremely lax and covered with scars and veins. With a patient who bruises easily, seeds are better.

I especially like the baxie points for patients who have trigger finger or other problems of contracture. While placing needles, it helps when we hold the patient's hand steadily in our own to avoid displacing hyperflexible joints. What matters in choosing these points is that the practitioner has a good feel for how well the hand and finger joints are functioning. Some patients have extremely tight hands and to loosen the joints may backfire and cause rebound hyperflexibility elsewhere. Bafeng, like baxie, is exceptionally useful to treat local pain and for treating plantar fasciitis and tarsal tunnel. Generally, a good sense of where the pain begins is gathered by knowing what the patient's feet feel like when they first get up vs. how things are by evening. How much do the joints loosen over the course of the day? These points are also useful for treating patients who lack proprioception.

The magic point for MCAS is baichongwo and if I had to pick one Extra point and only one, this would be it. My point location teacher, Dr. Shen, explained (and I wrote in the margins of my Deadman *et al.* text), "a patient with abdominal pains may well have parasites." Dr. Shen's commentary reminds us that Gu syndrome may be a factor in some of these presentations. If so, this point has extra resonance. Because I am always experimenting and trying to find ways to disperse Wind and Heat in the case of MCAS, I return again and again to baichongwo. Lanweixue can subdue Wind and Heat in an MCAS treatment. Relaxing a nodule at lanweixue followed by needling baichongwo can be effective. A good point prescription in this scenario would probably also include DU-24 and GB-20.

Point selection does require factoring in location and not just indications. It might be the best point in the world, but if it disrupts tendons or ligaments, it is not a good point. If the point is wonderful but sets off a rebound, as in the case of extraordinarily tight joints that will suddenly revert to being extraordinarily flexible (this you will see in patients over the age of thirty-five who were rubber bands until their early thirties and who then became what, in the common parlance, are known as "stiff bendies"), then it's not a great point. Especially when we treat a lot of hEDS, we will eventually become comfortable deciding where to experiment and where to start and stay very, very conservative. Patient comfort levels and confidence in us, their practitioner, are key.

Having a great point combination also requires knowing how to engage with these points. Acupuncture is not always the first or best choice. In chapter five, consequently, I address different modalities and how to choose them for the benefit of our esteemed HCTD patients.

## III. Palpation and the Fascial Planes

This chapter began with an outline of the ways in which the tangible body is delineated in written record. Its center pertains to the organs, their assigned meridians, and discussion of selected relevant points. And what of our inner wrapping? What of the fascia and the fascial planes? Western biomedicine has relatively recently become considerably more interested in fascia, and contemporary research in Chinese medicine has contributed to the building of knowledge surrounding this fabric. Knowing this tissue in more than one language and having the ability to read it through the lens of an hEDS patient's needs are valuable skills indeed. The intent of the final section of this chapter, consequently, is to invite critical and comparative thinking on the subject of fascia and HCTD treatment via Chinese medicine.

Biomedicine's inquiry into the nature of fascia is comparatively recent. The second edition of *Fascia: The Tensional Network of the Human Body: The Science and Clinical Applications in Manual and Movement Therapy* (2022) (hereafter *Fascia*), edited by Robert Schleip, Carla Stecco, Mark Driscoll, and Peter A. Huijing, is an excellent desk reference. Reading it alongside classical and strictly Chinese-centered resources is useful and instructive, especially since awareness of fascia's vibrancy is a prideworthy element of our practice in Chinese medicine.[15]

What becomes worthy of notice in medicine, be it Chinese or Western, shifts in response to cultural and economic factors, to be sure, but in this case—as with genetics—current interest in fascia was inspired by the ability of contemporary research's capacity to see at a greater level of detail. The introduction to *Fascia* begins by declaring in all caps, "WELCOME TO THE WORLD OF FASCIA!" (Schleip *et al.* 2022, p.xvii). Its author places fascia by noting that, "As every medical student knows and every doctor still remembers, fascia is introduced in anatomy dissection courses as the white packing stuff that one first needs to clean off in order 'to see something'" (*ibid.*). The author notes that this is no longer so, pointing to research papers appearing in peer-reviewed journals and the first International Fascia Research Congress held in Boston, at Harvard University, in 2007. Conferences in Amsterdam (2009), Vancouver (2012), Washington (2015), Berlin (2018), and Montreal (2022) followed. It is gratifying to note that the introduction of *Fascia* explicitly mentions Chinese medicine when pointing out that, "Hypotheses that accord myofascia a central role in the mechanisms of therapies have been advanced for some time in the fields of acupuncture, massage, structural integration, chiropractic, and osteopathy" (*ibid.*).

The chapter "Fascia and Traditional Chinese Medicine" references treatment via the fen rou, or tissues between the muscles; according to Ling Guan, this, "place of treatment is the *inter-flesh*, which is fascia" (2022, p.621). Dr. Guan notes that, "Some classical acupoints, such as GB34, are featured by fascia. TCM considers it to be the place where fascia meets and helps to treat systemic fascia diseases" (*ibid.*, p.620). He points out that the scalp is an area of concentrated fascia and remarks that when the needles are placed under the skin and above the muscles, "This area is called the Fen Rou of traditional Chinese medicine, and it corresponds to the space of human fascia—connective tissue" (*ibid.*, pp.620–621). Dr. Guan concludes by noting that, "Although ancient Chinese doctors did not describe fascia as accurately as we do today, or because of ancient language, we are not able to fully understand what they meant. It is clear that they were aware of the existence of this structure in the human body and found ways to adjust it functionally" (*ibid.*, p.624).

A contemporary description of fascia holds that, "A fascia is a sheath, a sheet, or any other dissectible aggregations of connective tissue that forms beneath the skin to attach, enclose, and separate muscles and other internal organs" (Stecco and Schleip quoted in Schleip *et al.* 2022, p.xix). Within the context of approaches to identifying and treating HCTD and hEDS, the fascia and fascial planes are of central importance. When we address the fen rou of the body and alter its relation to certain realms, points, or structures on that body, we shift our patients' experiences with their bodies and their pain.

To do so—to become expert—it is inevitably useful to return to the scholarship of practitioners in China. An invaluable resource for consideration of this subject is once again Wang Ju-Yi and Jason D. Robertson's *Applied Channel Theory*. It bears repeating that Dr. Wang is yet another Chinese physician who cautions against searching for specific points in order to treat specific diseases. He further states that, "Looking over China's vast medical tradition, one often finds that those who developed a more rigorous understanding of channel theory were also those who made the most lasting and clinically useful contributions to the field" (Wang and Robertson 2008, p.xv). In my estimation, practitioners who adhere to this philosophy will best be able to navigate advances in the study of fascia. Channel theory brings the study of fascia to life. So do excellent palpation skills.

Dr. Wang reiterates, as I do, the importance of palpation, declaring that, "the first goal of palpation is not to find points for needling, but to find clues about the state of organ function. Palpation should be thought of first as a diagnostic tool and only later as a tool for finding appropriate points for treatment" (*ibid.*, p.39). Patients who live within bodies that never function "normally" might have a hard time discerning value in their subjective experiences. Their channels do not share this inability to parse out differences between "normal" and dysfunctional. The evidence will be there for the practitioner who knows how to palpate. As a diagnostic tool, anyone who aspires to a specialization in HCTD and/or hEDS absolutely and without question needs to be able to accurately read the body via their palpation skills.

To read the channels of an hEDS patient is to learn a new language. We rely on what we know from our original languages (those being the narratives of anatomy and physiology on the biomedical end and the channels and their interrelations on the Chinese medicine side). We use those. But EDS bodies have a language of their own, each one unique. We find that body's baseline normal and we choose our thread. We go from organ to channel to point and circle back yet again. Some points will yield excellent results; others, less so. We may start with the functional organ or a more classical view of the organ as an umbrella category or system. One practitioner will privilege the channel as conduit over the point-by-point approach; another will center points. But in a body whose connective tissue makes all its own rules, we keep in mind, always, that each reading is distinct, ever-changing, and unique. The where, then, gives way to the how, or to modality, as we shall see next in chapter five.

# CHAPTER 5

# At the Heart of the Matter

## I. Languages of Pain

"Whose body is this?" I ask, gesturing with an open palm that is inviting and supine. We are sitting at my desk, me on one side and the patient opposite so that she is facing me directly.

"This is my body," she replies, gesturing towards herself and placing her hands across her heart, protectively but with an air of pride at her own audacity.

"And what happens if the doctor wants to do something that you don't understand or that makes you feel uncomfortable?" We both know the drill; this is a rhetorical question. My hands are crossed, expectantly, and I am leaning forward, ready to hear a well-rehearsed answer.

"I get to ask questions and the doctor needs to listen to me respectfully and answer my questions." The patient says this confidently, and even now, after almost a year of practicing, she still says it with an air of marvel that this should be so.

"And then what?" I ask, ever the proud professor.

"I decide what happens to me because this is my body!" she announces, hands on her chest, back straight, eyes shining with pride at her own sense of accomplishment.

We smile at each other, and exchange a fist bump, and then

the patient gets up to go to the treatment area, where she will settle in happily and enjoy an acu-nap that will leave her feeling rested and empowered.

Some patients will have medical teams and feel like they are genuinely part of a squad. They go to one doctor after the next and leave the encounters with the sense that they appreciate their care providers and that these specialists listen to them, value them, and deliver the best possible treatment to them. Other patients, especially when they fall into the cracks of the medical care system, either due to being categorized as a medical mystery or, perhaps, deemed to have conversion disorder or told to lose weight, do not feel empowered when they are dealing with biomedical practitioners. Different people will respond in different ways to biomedical systems. If a patient comes to us with medical PTSD, we may be their primary source of support as they learn to become empowered participants in their own healthcare.

This patient is one who has not been treated well during her labyrinthine journey. Within the first fifteen minutes of her initial intake, I knew that I needed to teach her a new language, one that could assert that her body belonged to her. We started the practice that I shared above at about her third visit. It took months before she could sit up straight and look me in the eyes as she answered. Initially, I would ask the questions and she would answer in a timid, uptilted tone, as if supplicant, "It's my body?" and, "I get to ask questions?" and, "I get to decide?" Her face would turn so red that, even though we were masked to protect against COVID, the bitter wash of dark crimson was visible around her eyes and all the way up to her hairline. As she spoke, she would cower in her seat as though she expected a blow from heaven in response to her temerity. It took months of practice before she was able to say that her body belonged to her while remaining upright and certain.

This is what it can mean to be a patient with a chronic

condition or a mystery illness. I have had a number of patients to whom I have taught the language of boundaries and efficacy to be used at doctors' appointments. She is not the only one. This patient, though, touches my professor's heart more than any other. I will never forget how she would shrink down her chair as if trying to disappear as she practiced asserting that her body belonged to her and not to the doctors who poked at her and sent her from one specialist to the next. As political winds of change in the United States seek to contain women's bodies today, especially, I worry about patients who may find that their autonomy is curtailed not only by individual practitioners but also by federal and local laws. When I teach patients to say, confidently, "My body belongs to me," it is an act of will that each one of us must take to heart.

Whose body is this?

And when this body is a body in pain, or it is a body that betrays itself with repeated dysfunction and chaotic process, it is not enough that we teach our patients to have confidence in their ownership of their tangible selves. Often, we will be tasked with helping them to articulate their experience of pain. How is it that a patient might narrate their experience? How can we ask questions that will elicit the information we most need from them? Taking a step further, we might also consider how we might support our patients and nurture not toxic positivity but, instead, a sense of efficacy that brings a measure of peace or respite.

We learned the pain scale in my second graduate program. From one, being the least, to ten—unbearable agony—the pain scale is supposed to be a concise measure that provides stan-dardized information. We did not use the more complex McGill Pain Questionnaire. This multi-factorial assessment tool con-sists of a line drawing of a human form that the patient can use to indicate where things hurt, a numerical system to indicate degrees of pain, and a menu of seventy-two words that may be chosen to narrate the contours of pain. It can be challenging for any medical care provider, allopathic or otherwise, to determine pain levels, especially when suffering is unique to the individual and not easy to capture in words.[1] When the root cause of the pain is baked into their connective tissue, it is most healing of all to acknowledge it, treat it, and respect it but, also, to make it possible for the patient—for the person—to find strength via their own narratives. Everyone has their strengths.

How can we be present for suffering yet offer alternatives that do not rely on toxic positivity?

People with hEDS have a high tolerance for pain. A person learns to live with pain or they cannot function at all. It is a common topic in social media circles to deride the one-to-ten pain scale as not being anywhere near adequate for the needs of an hEDS patient. Practitioners who treat HCTDs will want to be aware that this population does not hold this assessment in high esteem and some view it as useless and almost insulting. When we conduct the initial intake, it affirms the patient if we acknowl-edge the limits of the one-to-ten scale and invite the patient to elaborate on their experience with this scale. If the patient is afforded more than one way to narrate their own experience, it gives them an opportunity to assert agency over how they feel. This is good for patients and it sets a tone from the beginning: this is their story, the practitioner understands that, and we are here together as a team.[2]

Biomedicine and its narratives constitute a culture, a language, a practice, a territory. We in Chinese medicine have ours, too. What brings us to the medicine, how we are shaped in our programs, the patients we see, and how the patients see us all create a culture. Navigating the landscape of HCTDs requires intercultural competency from all of us, patients and healthcare professionals alike. Sometimes, it can be helpful, if only for the sense of solidarity and mutual understanding, if the clinician also lives with the condition they treat. But that is not necessary.

When we do share the condition, we need to be a little more careful to guard against thinking that we "know what it's like" because, in reality, we do not. With or without sharing the condition, either way, we do need to teach ourselves to listen. A patient who has been ignored or gaslit or taught that nothing they say will be understood may derive some measure of relief just by hearing the practitioner say, "I'm listening."

At the same time, we also benefit from thinking about our own boundaries. When I am in the early stages of getting to know a new patient, I am mindful about how I train the patient to view their treatment time. This process is similar to teaching students how to work within a classroom period. Does the professor allow students to drift in during the first five or ten minutes of class while she stalls, and then get started once everyone has arrived? Or is she prepared and ready to start on time, thus signaling that class time is precious and not to be wasted? How much time will be spent on lecture and when will the students have time to engage with one another? By about the third or fourth class, students know the drill and conform (or not, but that's a different ballgame). The same goes for patients. We want to be present for them and we want to support them. However, if we teach them that the sole focus of the appointment is pain and anguish, then the appointment will become a place to go and a location within which the patient can dig into their suffering and stay there, supported, for an hour or so.

I think that is unhealthy for patients and for practitioners. Patients want a place where they feel safe, understood, and supported and we, the practitioners, want to provide this for them. We do this by being mindful, especially during the initial visits. When we elicit information about pain or trauma from the patient, we learn to listen carefully and respond in ways that make patients feel heard. We will most certainly avoid toxic positivity, which is a form of gaslighting. Patients do not need to be told how to experience their own suffering or given platitudes about how to live within their own bodies. But we do not want to train a patient to wallow, either. The languages of pain, when understood, and the experience of being truly heard, maybe for the first time ever, really, can lead to a healing catharsis. But what if the practitioner is not necessarily prepared for the emotions and experiences of a patient who lives with chronic illness and pain?

In the final section of this chapter, Languages of Power, I return to this theme. It takes self-awareness, language skills, and diplomacy to create a container for HCTD patients. When we take good care of ourselves, we are able to take good care of others. When we learn to navigate vulnerability, trauma, and tragedy with grace, we are able to be present in a healthy way for our patients. We are all human. Developing trust with a patient, holding space while they express their pain so that we can adequately treat it, and knowing how to shape the encounter and when to step back at the appropriate moments so that the appointment does not become a therapy session (or worse, a trauma dump that leaves both parties exhausted) requires practice. Learning this becomes easier and easier if one begins mindfully and with self-awareness.

We return to this subject at chapter's end. In the previous chapter, we considered location, or specific channels, organs, and points. In this one, we investigate modalities. Ways to treat also require an HCTD lens and there are a number of questions to regulate our choices.

Which of our many excellent modalities are most suited for an HCTD patient? How can we plan and deliver them as filtered through the lens of HCTD? Most important of all may be the question of whether or not the practitioner needs to be well versed in all of our modalities in order to feel confident and empowered.

Where we find our confidence and conviction that yes, we are doing enough, also factors into the how-to equation that follows.[3]

# II. Modalities and Methods

## Acupuncture (and Equivalents)

Treating hEDS patients offers us a golden opportunity to become creative, responsive, and knowledgeable practitioners. We graduate from our programs with an extensive range of point prescriptions that we may use, from the standard to the esoteric. A patient with an HCTD will benefit from them the same way that someone without dysfunctional connective tissue would. That ST-36 is an excellent point is not a question. When treating for shen disturbance, we can rely on yintang. A person who comes in with prolapse will likely be on the table with a needle placed at DU-20 as part of the prescription. We do not needle deeply and perpendicularly when puncturing LU-1 and 2. And so forth. These things do not require discussion in this book. However, it bears repeating that the hEDS body has its own expression.

There is a difference between acupuncture treatment and acupuncture treatment for a body with an HCTD. We keep in mind that there are several ways to approach acupuncture point stimulation that will elicit de qi but which do not require acupuncture needles.

An hEDS body shifts, either due to ptosis internally or because the external flesh is tight and weak at one appointment and soft and loose at the next. We never can assume that a particular point will be the appropriate one until we palpate. With practice, it is not too challenging to learn which points might overwhelm a hair-trigger autonomic nervous system and to employ them judiciously. A good strategy is to slowly and gradually and consistently give the patient an opportunity to relax into the treatment and make incremental improvements.

When choosing a point prescription, we start by considering where the point is located. Needling into joints and disrupting dysfunctional tendons and ligaments is not wise until we know how the patient will react. Using thinner needles and being intentional, more so than normal, is a good strategy.[4] At least at the beginning, asking for feedback after the insertion and removal of the needle can be smart. Once we have established that KD-8 or other like points do not set off an unwanted cascade, then it is possible to confidently use them as long as we remain attentive. As the patient's body changes position, the weather shifts, or other things occur (MCAS flares, hormonal fluctuations), those points might not be as safe as they were at one time and we always want to be aware of alterations in the patient's stress or pain levels before needling into any areas that might be vulnerable. Some days, a point prescription will be unremarkable. Other days, if the patient is suffering a flare-up, what was an inoffensive needle makes the whole channel burn and ache.

As we are looking to determine point location, we pay attention to ptosis, both internal and external. Genuine understanding of how patients experience internal ptosis is a lesson. When I was newer to hEDS, I had patients who would become very distressed at their perception that their kidneys were moving around in their body cavity. They went to numerous allopathic physicians and had a number of tests, but nothing came of them and their distress was compounded by the aggrieved sense that they had been gaslit. At the time, I hadn't quite enough experience with ptosis so I did not know what to say, other than to promise never to needle BL-23 or any abdominal points that they found alarming. I didn't know what to do other than be sympathetic and compassionate.

Now, though? I look back on my earlier patients and recognize that I had not seen enough people with this complaint to understand that yes, it exists and no, MDs don't always catch everything. Time, seeing more patients like this, and my social media groups have convinced me that being able to feel one's organs floating about is not as rare as might be implied and that just because the MD does not find it doesn't mean that it's not real. When a patient tells me this now, I reassure them that they are not fanciful and that what we call Spleen qi sinking would be categorized as ptosis by Western medicine. Whatever term a person uses, it is real and it can be distressing. With that agreement in place, we then work towards finding points or other modalities that can tonify the Spleen and boost the qi without unduly alarming the patient. Just by listening and by responding with respect and empathy, we are healing a wound that our patients may have been carrying for years, if not decades.

It may be shocking to find out just how much a light stimulation can cause such a strong response in some patients.[5] It helps to know which areas tend to be exceptionally reactive. Especially with more sensitive people, the use of ear seeds rather than acupuncture needles can be sublime. In my clinical experience, SJ-5 and LI-6 can be sites of pain and subsurface Dampness and Cold, for example. If we roll our fingers gently down the arm, the place where a slightly gummy puffiness ends generally will be at SJ-5. Tapping our fingers upward, we may find a soft, gummy place at LI-6. This is very subtle to the fingers of the practitioner but even light stimulation reverberates astonishingly through the patient. We can go a half cun past SJ-5 towards the wrist or a half cun towards the radial and a half cun to the ulnar side of the gummy spot, and these are places to set ear seeds. Tap them gently into place and needle the legs or scalp. This promotes a moderate response that does not overwhelm the patient.[6]

My clinical experience with ear seeds is extensive. While still in my program yet already certified to practice tui na, I used ear seeds as part of my treatments because they are not insertive (thus requiring a license, as is the case with acupuncture). I also once participated in an event at a local resort. A group of about fifty travel agents who took care of big-ticket clients (touring musicians, important executives, and other similar) attended an event curated for rest and healing. The agents went from one area to the next to get massages, try sound therapy, experience aromatherapy, and more. I placed ear seeds on forty-six clients within a four-hour period. This was illuminating. About a quarter of them were mildly or not responsive. About half had a moderate response (typically, they reported feeling relaxed). About a quarter of them shifted their energetic field to the extent that even others in the room could see the effect. These people told me that they had never felt such a strong burst of calmness and focus in their lives, or that a place that had been painful for a long time had suddenly resolved, and other similar anecdotes. It was remarkable to see the range of responses in this group.

My clinical experience is that seeds are not a panacea (but what is?) but that they can be extremely useful no matter the outcome. For some people, ear seeds work. For others, at the very least they don't overwhelm their system. The combination of needles and seeds, especially for patients who have weak constitutions and extreme reactivity, is invaluable.

We want to learn to work with what our patients offer us and we learn how to deliver treatments that are safe for that person's unique hEDS body. And each of us has particular talents. Myself, I am not exceptionally talented with scalp acupuncture, but the scalp can be a safe place to needle as long as the practitioner avoids the occiput. Though I do not practice esoteric forms of healing, I think it would be enjoyable for patients to have healing mineral treatment with crystals and other stones that are placed on areas that might instead take ear seeds. I have done some work with the laser pointer in place of acupuncture needles and found it useful but that's not a particular skill of mine. In the hands of someone who really had a feel for lasers, they could be tremendously useful for hEDS patients.

One of the greatest gifts we get from treating hEDS is that doing so invites creativity. A treatment that works for tight muscles or Spleen yang deficiency or any other syndrome that we know well will work for an hEDS patient...and it almost certainly will work better with revision. We can always be eager to learn. Our patients benefit from this and so do we.

## Tui Na

Tui na is not only a method of healing. It is also a bringer of lessons. Though not all practitioners have the resources to study tui na, or the interest, it is a crucial skill for treating patients with hEDS. We learn volumes simply by touching with listening fingers. A practitioner who is not comfortable with touch may not be the best resource for patients with connective tissue disorders for this reason. Finding one's own language of healing touch, preparing one's practitioner self for treatment, and learning how to approach a body that has been in pain for a long, long time are skills to cultivate. Whether or not a practitioner chooses to offer tui na is a personal choice. However, we at least want to be familiar with this venerable healing practice and, for sure, we will focus on channel theory and palpation skills if we do intend to build a practice that supports HCTD patients.

Every hEDS body is different and each patient has lived within this body for some time. By developing excellent palpation skills and vividly nuanced listening hands, we can hear the words that the patient says and learn to connect what they mean as expressed by their particular body. At the time of this writing, I have been practicing tui na for almost a decade. There is still a new lesson every day as I develop my knowledge of tui na. I expect that this will be so for the rest of my career. Palpation, I believe, is a way to listen.

What we are listening for, when we read the body this way, are the different variations possible in a body that does not process collagen correctly. There is no norm. There is no average. There are not two or three models that a practitioner can study. Each and every individual is different and, not only that, their differences shift from one day to the next. A practitioner might do an excellent job of getting the trigger toe to relax only to find that another joint has seized up in an attempt to compensate for the newly achieved relaxation of the toe and ankle joints. Learning how to shift the balance just enough—not too much, not too little—takes practice. My clinical experience is that the fascial layer often feels cold and inert. By using light touch to begin, and focusing on warming from surface to inner layers, I am often able to get the patient's body to work with me, and that is the safest way to approach an hEDS body: with consent and in steps.

The techniques that work especially well with hEDS bodies include: rolling technique (gun fa) with the tips of the fingers, especially in lieu of spine pinching (nie fa). Rubbing with the flat of the palm (ca fa) with the intent to warm the channel on larger areas is also good, but the practitioner will want to ground themselves so that there is not too much pressure and not too little. HCTD fascia has much more give than non-HCTD tissue and it takes practice to learn depth of pressure with our hEDS patients. We practice. We learn to feel fascia by palpating for our own, and that of friends and family. Practice makes perfect. We keep trying.

Scalp tui na is often heavenly for patients. So is tapping along any cold and gummy channel to wake it up and warm it so as to reduce pain and anxiety. Gently, gently placing a facial rejuvenation cup and lightly popping it off a newly warmed channel can encourage a free flow of qi that would not be achieved without such coaxing. Warming the soles of the feet with the palms of our hands can open the Kidney channel and bring the qi of the Bladder, Gall Bladder, Stomach, Liver, and Spleen to the surface.

Whatever we do, we start with a moderate intent and an inviting stance. Qi will come to us if we ask nicely.

The strategy that works best, I find, is to first warm the channels and then see the response. Is that enough for the patient for the day? Is this someone with MCAS whose body responds vociferously to even mild changes in the force field? Well then. We can warm the channels, place some seeds on the points where we might normally needle, and let the patient take a little nap. We of course remember to give the patient plenty of time to get up from the table and adjust to being on foot, especially if they have POTS. At the next treatment, after getting the patient's progress report, we might warm the channels and see about adding some needles on the lower limbs in places that have larger muscles. How did that go? Eventually, our patient's body gets trained to relax in our presence and to not resist changes wrought by treatment. This takes maybe two or three treatments, though a small number will never learn to relax entirely. But we meet the patient where they are and celebrate their wins, no matter how large or small these steps forward may be.

I believe in preparing myself mentally to treat patients with tui na. I am a sensitive person and many hEDS patients are neurodivergent or otherwise highly sensitive as well. It is my duty to approach them with calm and gentle intention. So often, a patient has things done to them. When we treat a patient via tui na, we can try to step back from the mentality that we do to them. Instead, we might approach the body and invite it to share with us so that we do with, not to, a body that tends to be resistant. We respond in kind with appreciation and good listening. In so doing, we initiate a dialog between our hands and their joints. Their joints will tell our hands what they need to know, their scalp will speak, the soles of their feet will whisper secrets to us.

Our hands should say, in return, "Thank you for your trust, and is there anything else you would like to tell me today?"

## Cupping and Gua Sha

Cupping pulls and gua sha pushes; ultimately, both modalities are used to enhance circulation, release tension, move lymph and other body fluids, and supplement or restore a beneficial flow of qi. How these modalities work with an hEDS body is yet one more instance of "it depends." There are few hard and fast rules when addressing contraindications resulting from an HCTD and its comorbidities. But that should not be cause for avoiding cupping or gua sha. As we have been doing throughout this book, we simply need to approach this as a topic to be viewed through a certain lens, one that takes into account the needs of a body constructed by altered connective tissue.

The very simple, easy consideration to remember is whether or not the patient has MCAS or other sensitivities. If a patient is a bit sensitive to smells, putting oil on their body might suddenly make them *extremely* sensitive to smells. Before putting any oil on a patient, we ask them to smell it first. If this is not a super-sensitive patient, then it is probably safe to move right to treatment. If the patient is sensitive, the next step after having them smell the oil is to try a patch test. We can put a bit of oil on a spot of skin and leave it there while the patient rests during an acupuncture treatment. This has the added benefit of easing patient worries about undue reaction. Slowly but surely, we build trust and the capacity to experiment with treatment modalities. Taking all the steps is a good thing, even though it might seem obsessive at first.

We do wish to be aware of vascular fragility when we consider whether or not to include cupping in our treatment plan. A patient with spongy, very soft skin and lacy blue veins may not be the best candidate for cupping. What we can do, if we do feel that cupping is in the patient's best interest, is to use the more delicate glass facial cups and pop them on and off gently, rather than slide them. The medium-sized ones that run one-and-a-half inches across the diameter of the cup are useful for larger muscles, and the very small, one-inch ones, generally used for around the mouth or eyes, can do wonders for an hEDS body's paraspinal muscles. Placing the cup, popping it off immediately, and then rubbing the tissues between thumb and fingers is simple and easy. It also will have the same effect as a vigorous round of sliding cupping would on a non-hEDS body.

With respect to gua sha, I use either a jade instrument or the edge of a porcelain spoon rather than a metal tool. Less is often more when it comes to an hEDS body. My experience with trigger fingers and toes is that gua sha, rather than direct needling of the sinews, is effective. By softening the muscles and their attachments with a combination of gua sha and tui na, it is possible to disperse Wind and warm the channels without causing undue pain to the patient in the case of tenosynovitis.

With either modality, we decide how we will work around joints vs. what we might decide to do on areas of larger muscle. As a person with hEDS ages, they may end up becoming stiffer and stiffer. "Stiff bendies," as we are called in common parlance, can benefit from more vigorous cupping and stronger pressure with a gua sha tool, but the practitioner needs to palpate their joints first. If the tissue surrounding the joints feels crackly, thin, and weak, that is a sign to be gentle. If the patient has a particular joint that has subluxed regularly or frankly dislocated, it is smart to tread lightly with that joint. Every patient is different. Taking note of atrophic scars and relative thickness of the tissue will give a practitioner a lot of information. I personally do not like leaving my hEDS patients with notable marks after treatment; to me, if I have done this, it means that I am not being as careful as I should be. But a patient with larger, thicker muscles may benefit from stronger application. When we know our patients well, we know how vigorously (or not) to apply manual treatment.

The how, or technical application, of treatment is but one consideration. We also will want to weigh out the why, or treatment principle, at play. One of the characteristic aspects of HCTDs that we will soon come to know pertains to outcomes of poor circulation in relatively weak tissue. We see this in patients with thin skin, a slightly crunchy subsurface, and pockets of edema or vaguely sludgy-feeling fascia. Areas of the body that are fatigued, like the forearms or the calves nearing the knee, will display such textures. These areas respond very well to gentle cupping or gua sha. Moving the body's qi and fluids this way when the body is not capable of doing so on its own is soothing for patients. Once the practitioner has seen and treated even just a few different hEDS bodies, it becomes easy to determine where to make use of these modalities and to what degree of vigor to apply them.

## Let There Be Light: TDP and LED

People with hEDS tend to run cold but a dysautonomia presentation can go either way. Some people will suffer from hot flashes or fluctuating temperatures while others will experience the opposite and register three temperature variations: cold, colder, or freezing. While thermal design power (TDP) and other heating lamps have been widely used by practitioners of Chinese medicine, a relatively more recent surge in the popularity of light-emitting diode (LED) lamps is also changing how we deliver light therapies in our clinics. The therapeutic application of heat and light does have specific considerations when treating people with HCTDs, and these relate to safety and to particular approaches that will reap maximum benefit for hEDS patients. Both the TDP lamp and the LED source are excellent for these patients as long as we filter our use and expectations of them through the lens of connective tissue disorder.

When we use heat or light therapy with our hEDS patients, we get in the habit of noticing even faint changes in skin color.

It is not uncommon to see a lacy, mottled pattern on the lower limbs of both HCTD and younger women patients. We might also see it on a person's back. A reaction to cold, the mottled appearance of the skin should resolve once the person becomes warm. The term to describe this is *livedo reticularis* (LR), and causes of it are attributed to malfunction of blood flow at the surface of the skin or possibly blood vessel spasms. This is unremarkable in children and younger women or if it dissipates when body temperature rises. However, these patterns can be indicative of autoimmune disease, infection, or diabetes. A practitioner who routinely treats CTD and HCTDs learns to read this bodily sign after seeing both the benign and the concerning manifestations of it. The lacy purple of this corporeal sign is telling. If it does not dissipate in response to warmth then it more likely than not merits referral to an MD.[7]

In my clinical experience, the TDP lamp is more efficacious than one that simply heats the body. Stimulation from the heated mineral plate can increase microcirculation and soothe soft tissue. The lamp itself produces far infrared (below visible) light, which also compounds this effect. The expected outcome is increased and more effective blood circulation and stimulation of innate healing processes. When we treat hEDS, we want to get maximal effect via minimal stimulation of unstable joints. We might achieve this goal by combining TDP lamp therapy and other modalities. Warming a patient's sacrum or upper back with the TDP lamp and then palpating the area for relative warmth or coolness is instructive. There may be areas that become heated, as expected, and little patches that are cold, even after treatment. Running cups gently across these areas or using a pinching or rolling tui na technique can even out the warmth, thereby easing pain and encouraging healthier function. We can also invite the free flow of qi, if not de qi, by tracking how the body responds to targeted warmth and needling accordingly.

An LED-light therapy treatment can be similar; first, we apply the light therapy and next, we see what happens and direct qi in response. LED therapy is typically used by dermatologists and estheticians to promote healthier skin and improved collagen. In an earlier iteration of this modality, research by NASA scientists looked at how it promoted wound healing and cell health in astronauts. We are not able to stimulate the growth of healthy collagen via LED lamps. We can, however, use them the way we would a TDP lamp as described above. My experience with LED lamps is that they are exceptionally useful for patients who are constipated due to dysautonomia. Dampness that we would normally treat via SP-9 as part of a larger acupuncture point combination responds extremely well to the LED lamp on the bent knees as part of said treatment.

Each practitioner will want to experiment with both TDP and LED, but their ability to prime the treatment's effect makes it easier to be gentle and efficacious with patients with fragile skin and loose joints.[8]

## Nutrition and Herbal Medicine

Each practitioner will be different, and if nutrition is an appealing topic, then there is a lot we can do within this realm. It does require considerable specialist knowledge to deliver safe, effective nutritional education and/or therapy, especially if the patient has MCAS.[9] Especially if we focus on the Spleen/Stomach or ground our treatment in the principles of the Earth School, or if we are fascinated by current research pertaining to the gut microbiome, we are inclined to make food and healthy eating a priority in our patient guidelines. If so, we will want to be aware of the most pressing factors in terms of nutrition and hEDS. Even before we begin to think about the energetic properties of food, we need to consider a number of adjacent topics, including what role food plays in the individual's health history and wellness goals; how they view food and eating; and whether or not they are food sensitive or have MCAS.

In an ideal scenario, the practitioner is entirely fat neutral. Ideally, our attitude about weight looks something like this: we are interested in the patient's experience and we practice non-attachment about body size and shape. Orthorexia might be a concern. An individual who has very little agency regarding multiple aspects of their body may see food as one thing that is under their control. Someone with MCAS may need to severely limit and endlessly check what they can and cannot eat. In my experience, patients with orthorexia can be meaningfully helped by a therapist who specializes in disordered eating. It may be beyond our scope of practice to overly engage with orthorexia.

What about cultural baggage surrounding food? It may be hard to change a diet if the patient's family isn't entirely supportive and if they don't have the financial or other resources to do so. Selecting food based on what a person likes to eat due to their culture and history is important, too. When we have an idea of the cultural backgrounds of our patients, we can suggest foods that are nourishing for the Spleen that they will actually eat, or answer questions about foods that dry Dampness in ways that make sense. We will counsel that the patient avoids sugar; how, then, can a patient substitute and enjoy an occasional treat? What about food that helps people with chronic constipation? We want to remember that sweeping dietary change is not easy for anyone, much less a person who lives with chronic pain. Educating ourselves about our patients and their challenges helps us to offer nutritional support that is actually helpful.

If we opt to include herbal medicine into our protocol, it is prudent to begin with simple, well-known formulas like Si Jun Zi Tang (SJZT). As with BZYQT, this formula can be used in the instance of middle Jiao deficiency. Especially when used in low doses, SJZT combined with BZYQT can be safe and effective. In a contemporary form of modification, probiotics can be part of the program, though it is crucial to check for lower-histamine ones before suggesting them as an adjunct to our esteemed Four Gentlemen.

Nutrition education and herbal medicine are logical approaches to hEDS wellbeing. Contextual factors and our own interests will help us to decide whether or not we will choose to include these modalities in our practice. Especially when MCAS is part of the picture, there is a *lot* of extra learning involved if we wish to do so, and patients will often have a nutritionist assigned to them by their gastroenterologist. Though Chinese medicine is exceptionally useful in the realm of nutrition and herbs, we may decide to focus on one or another modality and feel satisfied with it...and we will be right. Acupuncture and/or seeds alone, or manual therapies, can be quite enough to effect meaningful change for our patients.

## Healing Movement

I would like to repeat an important point for all of us to keep in mind. To wit: we should not feel as though we are required to do everything and be everything for our patients. We can provide excellent and valuable service simply by becoming skilled in one or two modalities in service of hEDS wellbeing. I (obviously) feel strongly about tui na, while another practitioner might have a true talent for scalp treatment or lasers. We all have our talents and we do not have to be perfect at everything.

However, when we work with HCTD patients, pain is a feature. Whether or not we involve ourselves in their exercise or other movement-based therapies is an individual choice on the part of the practitioner. A patient who comes to us for pain relief may or may not be working with a PT or have other support for healthy movement. Whatever we do, we should be aware of the various options for our hEDS patients. This way, we can offer knowledgeable feedback if they ask questions and we can, if we feel moved to do so, build a referral network. At the very least, a practitioner might want to have an idea of what HCTD patients are capable of and interested in doing in terms of movement. With this knowledge, we are more able to provide safe, healthy treatments for patients who do want (or need) to include movement in their program.

Broadly speaking, it is a safe generalization to say that

movement and some form of exercise is healthy for almost all bodies. However, when it comes to hEDS, there are caveats and contextual factors to take into account. We can be a good resource if the patient wishes to begin a program of healing movement. Our very foundation of practice is built upon notions surrounding balance and we acknowledge the benefit of not going to extremes. A patient may ask us about setting up an exercise practice. If nothing else, we can be satisfied with simply knowing what sorts of gentle movement can be helpful to a body in pain and a psyche that experiences turmoil. We might also be tasked with treating an hEDS patient who has injured themselves while exercising; this requires an understanding of how sports injuries present in an hEDS body. What are the options for counseling a patient, either because they have questions about appropriate exercise or they are dealing with the outcome of inappropriate experiments in movement-based therapies?

A simple focus on breathwork can be helpful for patients who suffer from ribs that slide out of place or who have very weak neck muscles and readily displaced cervical spines. Either setting a patient up on the treatment table so that they are stable and beginning their treatment with guided breathwork or encouraging the patient to go online to find instructive videos can be helpful. It does not take that much time or energy on the part of the practitioner, and yet, as a result, the patient can learn to check in with their own body and breath, which is a real trick for many people and especially valuable for someone with hEDS. It takes creativity and awareness to treat patients with dysautonomia, too. When we are able to help them to learn ways to self-regulate, we are doing a genuine service to their wellbeing. We do not need to spend a lot of time on this aspect of the treatment; even just bringing awareness to the topic can help a patient.

Qi gong and tai chi are within the purview of a Chinese medicine practitioner's knowledge base. Some of us practice, and all of us should at least be familiar with the precepts of, qi gong. There are studies that demonstrate the benefit of qi gong for fibromyalgia relief, and these findings can extend to hEDS in equal measure. As to tai chi? This can be a useful tool for body awareness and lack of proprioception. Even a patient who cannot move easily or well can benefit from either of these modalities. If a patient comes to us for acupuncture, we are not obligated to turn the session into a combination of needling and movement. What can be useful, though, is for a practitioner to have referral sources or online videos to suggest.[10]

Depending on where the practitioner is located, it might be easier to find resources via local yoga studios. This, however, is a tricky topic. If the patient is already familiar with yoga, it should not surprise us to hear that this patient was the amazing student in the yoga class who could perform every posture to its extreme. These patients tend to have old injuries from their yoga days or stiffened joints that finally rebelled as they grew older. Otherwise, it is not uncommon to have patients who will hold back a scream of frustration at the mention of the word, simply because the answer to chronic pain and anxiety is too often the clichéd question, "Well, have you tried yoga?" It is wisely diplomatic to ask the patient if they have any opinions about yoga rather than suggesting it; this way, they can safely say whether this topic is cause for annoyance rather than interest.[11]

I am reluctant to suggest specific yoga instructors unless I know them personally. In my estimation, we as practitioners of Chinese medicine probably are wise to step lightly and not make specific recommendations. What we can do without risking liability is to stick to facts. We can educate our patients about different types of yoga and explain which might be more or less safe and why, for instance. For example, Iyengar yoga instructors are required to have a specific and substantive training and they are tightly regulated if they wish to maintain their certification. What I like about Iyengar is the rigor of their certification process and the fact that there is a certain level of standardization in their fields.[12] I have had hEDS patients who are non-functional without their ongoing Pilates practice; with the right instructor, Pilates may be a better choice than yoga for certain patients.

Personal training can be great for people with hEDS. Otherwise, it is common for patients to undergo ongoing physical therapy. Trainers and PTs can be allies to the practitioner of Chinese medicine, they can be off our radar and not especially relevant to the patient case at hand, or they can be problematic for a variety of reasons.

Once, a patient asked me if I thought physical therapy was damaging to people with EDS and whether I was against it. I responded by saying that people who go to a PT and have an excellent experience generally don't come to me. There is no need to do so if their PT resolved their issue. Instead, I get the patients who have gone to physical therapy and been injured or badly treated. In addition, I'm not a fan of PTs who perform the so-called "dry needling." I have nothing pleasant or conciliatory to say about PTs who think that what they do is science-backed, evidence-based dry needling, while what we do is "energy work" or other similar. However, and this is the most important point: I cannot do everything. I've had patients who underwent pelvic floor PT (which has included dry needling) and had excellent outcomes. Other patients with unstable necks have gotten treatment from a PT that I am not qualified to deliver. So, I told the patient, there are a few caveats but no, I am definitely not against physical therapy, and yes, I am glad when we can all work together for the benefit of a patient.

Chinese medicine cannot do everything, obviously, and there are exceptional PTs and trainers who are often super specialists in hypermobile wellbeing. One realm where we might not have thought to look is the field of circus medicine, but these are the people who treat contortionists and these are the people who have a higher instance of hEDS within their ranks.[13] I also think that anyone in our profession who is extremely well versed in martial arts could learn from both this book and from circus medicine in order to put together an excellent program of Asian martial arts and HCTD wellbeing. There are a lot of creative ways to support a person with hEDS as they develop towards their best level of health. A team effort is usually the optimal one.

Strength training can be excellent for hEDS patients if they are careful and if they have exceptional self-knowledge. It helps to have a personal trainer who knows hEDS. My personal history is a testament to the effects of strength training. In essence, I grew up in gym culture. During my teens and twenties, I trained under the direction of roughly a dozen trainers who were also competitive bodybuilders. During my first graduate program, I worked in the gym as a weight room consultant. Two of my trainers during that time frame were Olympic athletes. I have spoken with PTs about my history and they have uniformly agreed that I safeguarded my joint strength by working out the way I did. Competitive bodybuilders train to look good in competition and this means targeted muscle building and focus on individual muscles as one constructs a visual whole. It's a mentality and a method that, if applied correctly to an hEDS body, can be useful.

During my second graduate program, I opted to become a certified personal trainer with the thought that I could earn pocket money by working with private clients. I do not usually train patients, but this is a helpful credential to maintain because I can, when warranted, help a patient with self-paced programming if the patient wants to start slowly and on their own. As a trainer, I have provided feedback to patients as they progressed through a well-known program created by the American PT, Kevin Muldowney, who is widely known for the eponymous protocol contained in his book *Living Life to the Fullest with Ehlers-Danlos Syndrome*.[14] If a practitioner is interested in strength training, there are ways to make it relevant to the Chinese-medical therapy regimen.

Some of my patients are avid horseback riders. Others gave birth to three or more children (and that is certainly an athletic achievement). Some people with hEDS are active in the gym and still others are competitive bodybuilders. I've had patients who played a lot of basketball. Despite the challenges posed by connective tissue disorder, it is possible to be an athlete with hEDS. But there is a range of ability and disability and it truly does help a patient to be aware of their boundary and not go too far beyond its edges. It helps when the practitioner understands and is able to support and enhance what the patient wants to do, or at the very least, is able to ameliorate the outcome and limit further damage. If the Chinese medicine practitioner does not know a lot about strength training or other forms of physical movement, that is just fine. A patient's doctor can set them up with a PT and then the responsibility for outcome is decoupled from Chinese medicine treatment, which is something to consider.

The bottom line?

We do not have to know everything and we do not need to do everything. It helps patients who can't do vigorous exercise when their practitioner supports them just as they are and gives them options. Maybe the only option is breathwork while supported with neck pillows and leg bolsters. It helps when we know that exercise, if mindfully practiced, benefits our patients. But all we need to know is how HCTDs affect a body's capacity for movement and how these conditions factor into specific pitfalls. All we need to do is know how to safely treat mishaps. That is a lot of knowledge. We do not need to become PTs or personal trainers. What we have as practitioners of Chinese medicine is quite more than enough as is.

## Beauty Treatments

Acupuncture and other modalities of Chinese medicine for beauty are becoming more well-known the world over.[15] Micro-needling with a handheld pen, which is similar in form to mechanized seven-star needle treatment, has risen in popularity with acupuncturists and estheticians alike. When we consider gua sha and facial cups and aesthetic tui na, we can take pride in the way Chinese therapies are becoming fashionable and well regarded. It is no surprise, either, that people with hEDS might wish to try the holistic magic of Chinese medicine for cosmetic purposes. We all want to look and feel our best, and a person who navigates the challenges of chronic pain and illness is no different. I have been asked on social media forums if I perform cosmetic acupuncture on hEDS patients, and if so, what the special considerations are. In a comprehensive resource like this book, I would be remiss if I were to overlook the topic of beauty and cosmetic treatments for people with HCTDs.

There are three considerations when one is deciding whether or not to provide cosmetic treatments to people with HCTDs. These are: what does the patient want? What is the patient's presentation? How can a practitioner strategize treatment so that the modalities and methods respond to the specific needs and wants of the patient in question?

There are numerous ways that a cosmetic treatment can be uplifting and beautifying. Patients may want to restore vibrancy to their faces, the same as any other person. They may want a scar revision treatment. People will ask about stretch marks and whether or not Chinese medicine can help diminish them. This is the surface want. An inner yearning may be simply the opportunity to pamper their skin or to do something fun and relaxing. Even though we cannot "restore collagen" the way most anti-aging treatments promise, we can still make a person's face glow with health. People with EDS know that their collagen is defective. They do not expect a cosmetic acupuncture treatment to change that. But we can help to relax tight muscles and mitigate traces of pain and worry on a face. Everyone appreciates being able to look and feel calmer and more centered. There are always things we can do to make a person feel relaxed and cared for and special.

When we listen to not just the surface ask but also to what may be in their hearts, we hear what really matters to the patient.

Knowing the patient's hEDS or HCTD presentation before even touching them is crucial. Contraindications to cosmetic treatments that involve many needles or the micro-needle pen include autoimmune conditions. To this, I would add MCAS. A person with MCAS may experience a potentially dangerous flare-up as a result of the treatment. A person with dysautonomia might also react very badly to overstimulation on the face. What we can do before micro-needling, if this is what the patient wants, is to try a patch test on the face with .18x8mm Korean hand needles. If the patient does not hyper-react to having eight or ten needles placed close together on their cheek, we might decide to proceed with nano-needling and see how that works for them. Depending on the reaction, the practitioner might decide that micro-needling is safe for that particular situation. If the person has MCAS, just as with autoimmune conditions, it is safest to avoid the micro-needle treatment in favor of a more conservative strategy that, for example, supports the constitution.

My experience is that patients with hEDS generally do not tend to have wrinkles. They will have sagging skin and perhaps stretch marks, even on the face. They may have atrophic scarring. None of these conditions are necessarily amenable to acupuncture. Micro-needling seems to restore the texture of the epidermis in my experience, and I have had my best results with clEDS (this is a presentation with very loose skin). I would never micro-needle the face of a person with MCTD, or Sharp's syndrome. If the patient has the dry, papery skin that implies more tissue dysfunction than just one, that is an absolute contraindication. Stretch marks are a challenge to treat on anyone and not always worth the effort or investment.

The treatment of scars requires considerable experience,

patience, and dedication. If a practitioner has never treated a scar before or has minimal experience with scar revision, it is best not to start learning on the scar of an hEDS patient.

Gentle cupping, a facial massage with a jade gua sha instrument, and/or an excellent aesthetic tui na treatment can increase blood flow through the tissues, move lymph, and invigorate qi. We can treat the constitution as we would with any cosmetic treatment patient. We will be careful about fragrances, oils, and serums until we know if our patient can tolerate them.[16] But once we are assured that the patient responds well to these accoutrements, it is certainly possible to create a marvelous treatment that includes soothing oils and other similar.

Everyone loves to feel beautiful and pampered. We do not need to micro-needle or otherwise be aggressive in order to make our patients feel and look their best.

## III. Languages of Power

To begin this chapter, I addressed our need to listen to our patients and to be able to hear them when they speak. This opening section concluded with a reminder that we also want to protect our own psychological boundaries. We train our patients, to a certain degree. When we shape expectations for what an appointment entails, we are healthier, safer, and more effective when we know how to diplomatically redirect a train of thought that focuses too heavily on trauma. The ability to address chronic illness from the perspective of not too much and not too little—toxic positivity is as damaging as an overemphasis on hardship—but with just enough space for the patient to express and be heard in a healing way is a skill to cultivate.

When I was in my first graduate program, we were required to take one class on pedagogy and we had a weekend seminar at the beginning of every new academic year. Nobody enjoyed these things. Most of us were in graduate school so that we could have research careers, and people who were too enthusiastic about pedagogy were either gearing up for their dissertations on second language acquisition or preparing themselves for a lifetime of not publishing and complaining about their colleagues who would actually publish. We probably all could have used a bit more instruction on pedagogy, though, and I was lucky to come from a teaching family. At least, as I learned to teach, I could ask my parents for insights. Most of my graduate student peers viewed asking for help as an admission of failure but, as the daughter of educators, I walked into Indiana University's excellent Teaching and Learning Resource Center confidently and with the expectation that they would help me (and they did).

I noticed a bit of this in my second graduate program. We had some coursework in topics related to case management, clinical communication, and mind-body theory but these were largely introductory. We were not trained to become psychotherapists. But would it have helped us to have more coursework, similar to that of a psychotherapist? I do not think so. I think we had a lot to learn in order to become excellent practitioners of Chinese medicine. And yet, in many ways, cultural expectations surrounding Chinese medicine as a holistic approach to wellbeing create the expectation that we do treat the psyche at this level. How, then, is a practitioner to acquire an appropriate level of skill in this arena?[17]

In the early stages of my second program, a visitor gave a brown-bag talk. He was an MD, a graduate of Harvard, and a certified health coach. At the time, I was working my way through a process to acquire this same credential. Listening to this MD speak about not having had enough coursework in communication while in medical school was instructive. His perception was aligned with mine, albeit for different reasons. Though I had nearly two decades' worth of teaching experience, I felt that learning the narratives of health coaching would be useful.

Teaching Spanish literature and culture is not the same as sitting down with patients, and I hoped to learn a new language via my health-coaching certification. And yet, it was startling to me to think that doctors would not have learned this in their programs. By the end of my second graduate program, I had treated enough patients to see the damage poor communication engenders. I did finally understand why that speaker had taken the time to become a certified health coach in addition to his MD. But at his brown-bag talk, I really was taken aback that a Harvard-educated MD would want to become a certified health coach.

Health-coaching certifications do not imbue a practitioner with medical knowledge (we get this from our graduate programs and complete that certification process via board exams and state licensing requirements). Instead, they create a type of listener that is skilled at helping a client identify and achieve health goals.

A practitioner of Chinese medicine who is (understandably) not too keen on the idea of adding yet more training on top of the years of work required to become an acupuncturist has options. My health coach certification program emphasized the trans-theoretical model of change set forth by James Prochaska and colleagues in the 1970s and still widely used today. This model looks at change as a series of stages that begin with precontem-plation (unawareness of the need for change or resistance to it), progress through steps that include contemplation (getting ready), preparation (ready), and action (actively doing), and conclude with maintenance (at six months without relapse). Success in the program meant demonstrating the ability to meet clients where they are and engage with them based on their stage of change. This is not the only way to work with people. Moti-vational interviewing is another technique used in healthcare settings as a way to help clients identify their needs and goals. Neuro-linguistic programming also offers a model designed to enhance mindfulness in communication.[18]

If we are interested, it is useful to become certified. We are able to work with health-coaching clients outside of our state through virtual visits and it is easier to get insured to provide this service when one has this credential. But it is not necessary. We do not need to become health coaches to learn about these and other useful models of communication. There are a number of online resources and books we can read if we are interested in honing our communication skills.

Languages of power do not only reside within the gift of diplomacy. We also become stronger practitioners and professionals when we identify our sources of knowledge. When Dr. Ching writes of intuitive knowledge in his excellent book, *The Art and Practice of Diagnosis in Chinese Medicine*, he is not referring to one's gut sense of things. Instead, he is writing of the kind of intuition that comes from a mature intellect, substantive clinical experience, and a willingness to continue studying.

As practitioners outside of China, especially when we do not speak or read the language, we expect to work harder if we wish to excel. Where do we get our knowledge and authority? Is it because we put forth considerable effort to learn how to conform to biomedicine's language, standards, and systems? Or do we rely on translations of classical scholarship? Is there a middle ground? Where do we find it? How do we identify it?

Finding validation in being accepted by insurance companies might not be useful for someone who works with HCTDs. Not all of the biomedical physicians who specialize accept insurance because complex diseases like hEDS and MCAS require more time than an insurance company will allow, and it is even less likely that an acupuncturist could get decent compensation for the amount of time we spend with HCTD patients. If we only look to Western biomedicine's terms for authority then our patients lose out on what Chinese medicine uniquely has to offer. If that is our choice then we might as well send them to PTs for dry needling or to a naturopath for supplements. Patients do not need us if we do not trust our own medicine and, instead, look to allopathic systems for validation.[19]

I have argued that Chinese medicine, when delivered far from Beijing, constitutes a borderlands practice with its own culture and identity. In concluding this chapter, I want to acknowledge what an exciting time it is to be a practitioner. I look at the excellent translating work that is becoming more and more available and am encouraged. There are practitioners and organizations who move easily between Chinese and Western medicine but who clearly privilege Asian medicine. In the face of HCTDs and MCAS, it is not a matter of the cliché of how Chinese medicine is great for things that Western medicine doesn't handle well, which brings with it the implication that we are picking up scraps from biomedicine's table. Instead, it is that we have substantive offerings, period.

Chinese medicine has techniques, modalities, theories, and practices that are uniquely beneficial for these chronic conditions. We are multicultural and multilingual, and we are rich in history and profoundly grateful to China, its source. When we speak in the language of Chinese medicine, we teach our patients about personal empowerment. We when speak it to each other and expect that other healthcare providers respect us for what we have to offer, we are also speaking a language of power, even if that language is not Chinese or the classical written words of venerated medical ancestors.

# CHAPTER 6

# Return Over and Again to the Clinical Experience of Others

## I. Traduttore, Traditore

To translate is to betray.

The Italian adage "traduttore, traditore" indicates just that: translator, traitor. Its origin harkens back to cultural rivalry between Italy and France when French translations of Dante's *Commedia* outraged the gatekeepers of the Tuscan dialect that would eventually become the standard for spoken Italian. Even now, the challenge of rendering one language's meaning and beauty and nuance into another invites discord. The classical discourse used to write canonical medical texts is not easily deciphered even by native speakers of Chinese languages. The saints who filter these texts through lenses of English or German or Spanish or any other language have their work cut out for them. But difficulty remains. How does one take a word, so laden with meaning in its original, and replace it with another that is flat and perhaps dull in comparison? How does a collection of words—a medical text either ancient or contemporary—convey the majesty or impact or crucial instructions of its origin? For the consumer of the translations, the clinicians who will turn to patients and translate, yet again, the question remains: how do we know if our translation is apt or if it is, instead, a betrayal?[1]

Lexical gaps, or absences of words that adequately convey the yang, or vibrancy, of the original when rendered into the yin, or substance, of the translated text, are remedied by adaptations, borrowings (as we do when we write the word *qi* or *zang* or *fu*), and compensations. We try, sometimes successfully and other times falling short, to find a shaoyang, or pivot. Our clinical experience grows and we return to our translations and deepen the connection to medical ancestors who are centuries removed or, in the case of those of us not Asian, not even truly our own.

What does the adage *traduttore, traditore* mean for a practitioner of Chinese medicine who works with heritable disorders of connective tissue? Even native speakers of Chinese might ask themselves this question, for hEDS is not a condition that we find in the *Shang Han Lun* or the *Nei Jing*. We all, in fact, may have occasion to ask ourselves how we honor Chinese medicine when treating diseases that are defined and largely regulated by Western biomedicine.

To answer this question as thoroughly as I might wish is another book in and of itself. A complete response begs for a lengthy digression on the subject of cultural competency, not to mention the postcolonial subject and other aligned topics. This is not the place. However, there is a shorter answer, one that fits into this chapter and its concluding invitation to further exploration of the many facets of medicine, culture, and chronic illness. To consider the matter of language acquisition and multilingualism and to apply it to this theme is, I think, a worthy first step in the thousand-mile journey that takes us to Beijing. The famous Sontag quote, "Everyone who is born holds dual citizenship, in the kingdom of the well and in the kingdom of the sick. Although we all prefer to use only the good passport, sooner or later each of us is obliged, at least for a spell, to identify ourselves as citizens of that other place" (1978, p.3) takes us even further.

We learn to navigate complex chronic illness, either in ourselves or in our patients, by critically engaging with the material and by learning how to read familiar texts with different lenses and ever-changing depths of knowledge.

As any student who remembers me will remember *very* clearly, I preferred to ask questions rather than to make declarations. Or when I did state this or that fact, or cite some or other text, I would ask questions. What about this? How about that? Critical thinking takes training and practice. No matter how smart we are or how well read, it is a skill to cultivate.

I have written elsewhere in this book that hypermobility and EDS, characterized as rare today, eventually will become widespread, similar to diabetes or long COVID. Biomedicine has much to offer these patients, both in terms of diagnostic technology and treatment modalities. Laboratory researchers will identify and name aberrant genes. Physicians will delineate best practices for the clinical encounter. Western biomedicine will fall short. Systems will overlook or marginalize. Patients will look elsewhere. Traditional Asian medicine, be it Chinese or other in this family, has worlds of wisdom and healing with which to not only fill in the gaps but also create new models. We, too, will fail our patients at times. We cannot do everything. But, as we say in Spanish, *cada olla tiene su tapa*, or every pot has its lid. Yes, this is a proverb used in the context of romance, but for a patient in desperate need of meaningful health solutions, there is an element of love when we find the modalities that work for us. I also believe that Chinese medicine is now firmly within a borderlands space, and so, in the case of hEDS, are our patients.

To navigate these interspaces requires curiosity, enthusiasm, and a willingness to think the way a comparative literature scholar does: critically and via comparison. The central aspect of this final chapter relates to cultivating interdisciplinary practices to nurture this project. Subsequently, I conclude this chapter with a provocative question. To wit: are we a melting pot or mixed salad? But once again, I am ahead of myself. Before we consider subjectivity, we must, instead, think about *books*.

## II. Interdisciplinarity, or Attending to Relations Rather than Givens

At about the time frame when this *Chinese Medicine* was in an embryonic stage, Lawrence Afrin gave a talk and subsequently published a paper that presented a novel theory. In his estimation, and given the failure to discover a genetic link to hEDS, Afrin posited that some manifestations of hEDS might be due to MCAS. This was in October 2021. As this book moved closer to its due date with my editor, new findings regarding methylation disorder and collagen expression were published.[2] This was in April of 2023. Four years ago, a fourteenth subtype of EDS was discovered. The gene alteration in question was found in only four individuals from three different families. Three years ago, one of my patients with a multi-systemic disorder that complicated their EDS presentation was found to have a novel gene mutation that was not reflective of EDS but, instead, related to yet another connective tissue dysfunction. Like most people who follow research trends, I expect that a genetic marker for hEDS will be identified in 2023 if not shortly thereafter. We are in a moment of discovery and proliferation.[3]

There is always something to learn. We must become excellent scholars of the human skeleton, the fascia, the muscles, the tendons, and the ligaments. We cannot help our patients if we do not know digestion and its discontents. We are called upon to become exceptional listeners and communicators. If we are lucky enough to not know HCTD via personal experience or to suffer from MCAS, we will need to work on our empathy skills. We need to become more versatile and committed as practitioners of Chinese medicine at the same time that we bolster our knowledge of Western biomedicine. It may seem fruitless to work with patients we have no hope of curing, but it is truly worth all the hard work doing so demands. And I do believe that more is coming. The Ehlers-Danlos syndromes, especially the hypermobile variety, will become relatively common within ten years, if not less, alongside the ravages of complex syndromes like long COVID and an increasing variety of autoimmune diseases.

How, then, to nourish one's study of Chinese medicine? For answers, I would remind of the anecdote of hand-copying passages that I shared regarding my first graduate program. I will also reference Wang Ju-Yi. Reading Dr. Wang's comments about his own process of knowledge acquisition brought back so many memories, and his words deeply touched my heart. "Return over and again to the clinical experience of others," he told his student, Jason D. Robertson (Wang and Robertson 2008, p.178). Reading these words is a call to arms for all of us.

Dr. Wang had his favorite resources that he selected after much discernment, and he shared this strategy with his student who then shares it with us, the readers. "After searching through many different texts and speaking with my teachers about their favorite books," he explains, "I settled on three favorite works and developed a study method based on those." His learning process was comparative and methodical:

> My strategy for using these books was as follows... I would first determine an organ-based categorization of the disease type using mainly differential diagnosis. Then I would see which points the *Classic of Nourishing Life* would recommend for treatment. I would next go to the sections on those individual points in both of the first two books and compare and contrast how the two books understood the functions of each point... This process gave me considerable insight into how great scholars

and clinicians from other eras understood the effects of the points on the qi dynamic. (*ibid.*, pp.178–179)

How we approach hEDS requires the same systematic approach. But a contemporary practitioner's context, whether or not we have access to source texts in their original language, requires that we incorporate resources from outside our traditions into our knowledge-acquisition project.

Selecting and critiquing a complete library is beyond the scope of this book but it is a worthy conclusion to end with a focus on particular resources that we, as practitioners, must know and can certainly use. How each of us builds our knowledge base as we develop treatment strategies for our HCTD patients is, in part, idiosyncratic. And yet, a canon of sorts allows us all to speak a common language.

What follows is a relatively short, yet valuable, guide to building an interdisciplinary knowledge base.

## The Ehlers-Danlos Syndromes

As practitioners of Chinese medicine, we graduate from our programs trained in a broad spectrum of diagnosis, etiology, and treatment principles. The methods with which we drain Damp or transform Phlegm or boost yang qi according to patient need do not radically change because the patient comes to us with an HCTD presentation. What does need to expand is our understanding of this hydra as it extends beyond our own parameters. This way, we return to the methods and principles we know so well and we shift their application to fit the needs of a very specific patient population. We do need to be familiar with hEDS culture and community and we are better able to serve this population when we can also place them within their biomedical context. To do so requires an encyclopedic knowledge of the *and what else?* of HCTDs.

First and foremost, a practitioner who wishes to be of service to HCTD patients must know that worldwide bonds connect us all. We of the HCTD community do have our own cultural connective tissue and it is strong. People with EDS and their loved ones are a force to be reckoned with on a worldwide scale. Social media communities, the EDS ECHO project, and entire volumes written by people who either live with this condition or are adjacent are living expressions of the determination and creativity that characterizes this sector.

Two encyclopedic resources that I now compare are exemplary in this regard.

*Disjointed: Navigating the Diagnosis and Management of Hypermobile Ehlers-Danlos Syndrome and Hypermobility Spectrum Disorders* (2020) is a collection of essays brought together and edited by the mother of a daughter with EDS. Diana Jovin gathered material from over thirty different practitioners and scholars, and the content of this volume begins with a history of EDS and covers diagnosis, comorbidities, treatment, legal ramifications, academic accommodation, lifestyle habits, and more. Though it mentions acupuncture in a brief paragraph on page 441, there is nothing of substance regarding Chinese medicine in this book. Even so, *Disjointed* offers an exceptional overview of EDS. The bibliographies at the end of each entry are useful. This is also a valuable resource because patients love it and read it. When a practitioner speaks knowledgeably of *Disjointed*, the patient gains confidence in the practitioner. If the patient has not heard of this book and we suggest it, the patient is usually happy and excited to learn of it.

The second encyclopedic resource is *Transforming Ehlers-Danlos Syndrome* (Daens and Dubois-Brock *et al.* 2022). This is not the fruit of a loving mother's efforts, as with the previous book. Instead, this is the work of a successful MD from Belgium who developed EDS as the result of a homophobic attack that not only acutely injured him but also triggered the expression of his EDS.[4] Herein, the reader will experience the substantive heft of a knowledgeable physician who has a significant emotional attachment to the material. Not only is his scholarly capacity demonstrated within this large volume. He also shares his heart within its pages. Dr. Daens co-founded GERSED Belgium, an EDS study and research group, and there is a version of this text in French. Being a voice for EDS became a vocation for this physician.[5]

This is also valuable resource. A reader is privy to European constructs of EDS when reading this book. While there is overlap with American scholarship, it is not the same. He does appreciate and speak well of acupuncture, which of course endears him to me as a reader. The author also shares excellent further resources for European research and, especially for speakers of French, this is helpful. For those who do not speak other languages, it is still good to know the names of European authorities in the field. It is extremely valuable for Americans to see the contours of European thought on this topic, just as—I am sure—it is useful for Europeans to see what physicians like Lawrence Afrin, Clair Francomano, Brad Tinkle, and others who are well-known names in the US have to say. We learn by reading each other's work. This book contains thorough and exceptionally valuable information for anyone who wants to engage with the material, and the cultural flavor of it makes this book a joy to read.

A practitioner who wishes to specialize in HCTD must, without question, read both of these books and should have desk copies of them for reference.[6] Our understanding of what both texts convey becomes enriched when we then return to our own medical tradition and reread our seminal volumes against the knowledge we have thus gained.

One of our most valuable resources will always be *Applied Channel Theory in Chinese Medicine: Wang Ju-Yi's Lectures on Channel Therapeutics* (Wang and Robertson 2008). We may read this book over and over, like an old friend, and feel as though we are directly learning from a teacher. Bodies whose connective tissues shift and slip and which are characterized by instability have a language of their own. A practitioner can spend many afternoons reading and rereading just the chapters on the taiyin and jueyin systems and then see, in one's patients, just what Dr. Wang outlines about the functions of the two organs that are so very important in the case of EDS; namely, the Spleen and the Liver. If we take to heart his exhortation to, "return over and again to the clinical experience of others" (*ibid.*, p.178), we will see every chapter in this book reflected in our patients.

Especially for practitioners who do not have a mentor or who were not fortunate to ever have had sustained connection with a master practitioner, *Applied Channel Theory* is also particularly valuable because its narrative structure invites the reader into a mentorship. Dr. Wang seems to love to teach and Jason Robertson frames his delivery of knowledge so that we, the reader, can share in his own learning experience. The clinical pearls contained in this book are numerous. But by reading the book with an eye for pedagogy, we also experience the process of learning in a meaningful way. As a former professor, I especially love this book for its teaching structure. As we learn to work with chronic and complicated illness, a guide such as this one is invaluable.

*Rheumatology in Chinese Medicine* (Guillaume and Chieu 1996) (hereafter *Rheumatology*), particularly when read alongside *Applied Channel Theory*, is invaluable. If I were teaching a course on this subject, the Translator's Foreword would be part of the assignment. The translator, David Vachon, notes that rheumatology is a traditionally French medical specialty and states that, "The translation of this book represents a delicate balance among ancient Chinese thought, modern Chinese medicine, the French acupuncture tradition and the American language and culture" (*ibid.*, p.xviii). This book is useful for its descriptions, case studies, and pattern identifications of CTD. When we read it alongside *Transforming Ehlers-Danlos Syndrome*, our horizons expand in part because these are both solidly French narrations. Though not as much now as initially, hEDS is within the purview of rheumatology and it is common for patients to have a rheumatologist on their healthcare team. The opportunity to deeply study this field as it pertains to Chinese medicine and emanates from its country of origin is invaluable.

Interdisciplinary reading requires more than just forays into comparative medical practice. For this reason, we return to Lorraine Wilcox's translation of *Categorized Essentials of Repairing the Body Zhèng Ti Lèi Yào* (Xuē 2017). Reading this book reminds me of the work I did for my Ph.D. minor in Art History. This project entailed a solid year of my life picking through *Le Ricordanze* (a record-keeping account) of an average working painter of Renaissance Florence, one Neri di Bicci. His workshop journal started in March of 1453 and ended in April of 1475; as with Dr. Xuē's records, the entries are succinct but redolent of history and of daily life. If memory serves me, the painter fixated on matters like having enough cloth while offhand comments brought to life his family and personal interests. With Dr. Xuē, we read of people who have been beaten and others who have fallen from horses. We read of real people who are genuinely hurt. Of a young patient, he says, "A child's humerus came out of his socket and was reinserted. He had swelling, pain, and fever. He took herbs to flow qì and so forth but the symptoms increased a lot..." (*ibid.*, p.79). Of course, I wonder why that child's joint dislocated and am relieved to read that he recovered.

These small portrayals of a life spent treating injured bodies are worthy narratives, and they are instructive, too, when set alongside *Applied Channel Theory* and *Rheumatology*. Reading how he used herbal medicine brings added life to formulas that we know and use today. Dr. Xuē specifically mentions Li Dong-Yuan in his accounts and this mention is accompanied by a translator's note explaining that, "Xuē Ji tended to favor his formulas and theories of treatment" (*ibid.*, p.38). Case study narratives bring Chinese medicine to life for contemporary readers and this particular book is especially precious for anyone who wants to work with bodies in pain.

And pain, for its part, is a constant in the treatment of hEDS patients.

## Pain

The presence of pain that has lasted for over three months is a box that the MD will check off when making a clinical diagnosis of hEDS. Harkening back to chapter two of *Chinese Medicine*, the topic of pain holds the same pitfalls as an initial appointment allowed too many tangents will have. In other words, it is possible to focus on pain, chase after pain, and get pulled into a vortex of engagement with pain that, ultimately, does not help the patient and can cause burnout in the practitioner. Patients in online forum discussions lament being fired by their doctor for being too complex and demanding for the physician's liking. I have never seen online chatter about being fired by an acupuncturist but I can imagine that it has happened. I can also readily picture an acupuncturist, especially a newly licensed solo practitioner, becoming thoroughly overwhelmed by the needs of a chronic pain patient. We want to help people, those of us in both Chinese and Western medicine. Engaging with chronic pain requires good boundary setting and considerable knowledge, both for the patients' sakes and for ours.

The aforementioned *Rheumatology* remains seminal. We have already established that it is a sine qua non for its contributions to our cultural and historical knowledge base. Within the context of pain, per se, this resource is further invaluable because it outlines all forms of Bi syndrome and their treatments. A practitioner who routinely treats for pain needs to essentially memorize this book. There are minimal references to Western biomedicine and what appears does so in the service of Chinese medicine. In the chapter on ankylosing spondylitis, for instance, the description of this condition is terse, consisting of five bullet points and a summary, "This disease targets young men between the age of twenty and thirty; there is a hereditary predisposition component, confirmed by the presence of the HLA B27 antigen" (Guillaume and Chieu 1996, p.175).[7] The rest of the section focuses on Chinese medicine's precepts and treatment strategies.

The introduction to Part Four of this treasure reminds us, maybe, that pressing and probing was overlooked in classical literature, and Guillaume and Chieu begin by stating that, "To our knowledge, there is no traditional Chinese medical treatise dedicated exclusively to rheumatology" (*ibid.*, p.303). However, the authors did the work of compiling relevant excerpts of translations for us, their readers. The entire section consists of classical sources and point prescriptions for rheumatological conditions. This is a book to read over and over again. In so doing, a practitioner will become steeped in the practical application of Chinese medicine and acquire a second language in rheumatology. Especially once fluent in the language of HCTD as well, we are then able to be of immeasurable service to our patients.

Rheumatology is a complex specialty. Chronic pain is complex. When we treat conditions that biomedicine cannot always resolve, it is especially incumbent upon us to be able to clarify what we are doing and why; often, we need to be able to define our terms in the other language, that of biomedicine. Holding *Rheumatology* as a primary text allows us to do this.

It is not enough to be cognizant of dysfunction (vis-à-vis close reading of *Rheumatology*). The tangible connection between practitioner and patient is most aptly served via, as I have argued, tui na. Anyone who specializes in the treatment of HCTD should become expert in this modality. That probably will not happen, but *The Practice of Tui Na: Principles, Diagnostics, and Working with the Sinew Channels* (Aspell 2019) brings sinew theory to life, whether or not we include manual therapy in our treatment plans. If I were teaching a course on HCTDs, I would require students to demonstrate mastery of all of the aforementioned resources on an individual level and show how, as a collection, they create a knowledge base necessary for treating hEDS. What the reader acquires from readings of *The Practice of Tui Na* can then be transferred to an acupuncture-only approach, especially if set alongside other valuable resources such as, for example, Callison's *Sports Medicine Acupuncture: An Integrated Approach Combining Sports Medicine and Traditional Chinese Medicine* (2019) if that focus speaks most to an individual practitioner's unique patient base.

There is a vast range of resources on the biomedical side if we are looking for a solid desk reference. *Kinesiology of the Musculoskeletal System: Foundations for Rehabilitation* (Neumann 2010) is a dense tome that thoroughly covers every facet of movement, from structure of joints to relation with peripheral nerves and more. Orthopedics and rheumatology are two areas that require extensive knowledge if we would wish to tread HCTD. Reading this book or others similar with great care makes our subsequent rereading of *Rheumatology* that much more fruitful. We need to know how a so-called normal body works in order to provide thoughtful care to one that tells its own story and marches (or slips out of place) to its own beat.[8]

At the same time, an interdisciplinary reading of pain acknowledges that the realms of science and medicine are limited. We must expand our horizons when we treat chronic pain and complex illness by setting aside, at least for a time, our textbooks and tertiary collections. *The Culture of Pain* (1993) by retired English professor, David Morris, is one of many potential resources for locating this sensation within a larger cultural framework. We will always remember that pain is more than the physical body. It is not just sensation that brings a patient to the clinical encounter. It is not just the purview of the nervous system, the brain, or the eyes that weep in response to its punishment. Pain is a language. It is a construct. It is a process and an unfolding. When we deal with pain, and if we are to deal with pain, we also need to expand our cultural awareness of it and engage multiple filters with which to assess and treat it.

Consequently, I argue with heartfelt passion for a reference guide to culture and pain, one to read alongside our books on kinesiology and trigger points and referral patterns. I argue less for anthropology, sociology, or history; instead, I think a literature scholar's perspective rounds out our inquiry most properly. Hence, *The Culture of Pain*. In it, Morris asks and answers questions about what pain is and how pain is voiced. He considers what history, literature, culture, biology, humor, sexuality, and deviance have to say about pain. Whether or not a practitioner enjoys this sort of reading is beside the point. What we gain from it is an expanded lexicon. Imbibing books like this and then circling back, once again, to *Rheumatology* or other seminal texts in Chinese medicine gives a richness to our engagements with patients. It teaches us to listen. We learn to critically think about pain in expanded ways when we fold this or other similar resources into our interdisciplinary roster.[9]

## Gu and MCAS and Lyme: Chronic Inflammation

Chronic inflammation as an umbrella topic warrants a multi-volume set of books; individually, Gu syndrome, MCAS, Lyme disease, post-Lyme, and chronic conditions like long COVID merit weighty tomes of their own. What a practitioner of Chinese medicine needs to know about this realm as it fits into the larger picture of HCTD treatment is that these are or will become the illnesses of our generation, and that we in Chinese medicine have potent arms with which to fight against them. As with any of the other facets of HCTD, the best defense is a knowledgeable offense. To that end, I recommend the following resources with the caveat that they are but introductions.

When we treat HCTD and/or MCAS, we develop a close bond with the work of Lawrence Afrin. *Never Bet Against Occam: Mast Cell Activation Disease and the Modern Epidemics of Chronic Illness and Medical Complexity* (2016) is required reading. It is a hefty tome that outlines one jaw-dropping case study after the next. We may not realize just how incredibly disabling chronic inflammation and aberrant mast cell activity can be. We learn by reading this book. Patients wait months and even years for an appointment with Dr. Afrin and he sees the most puzzling and complex cases imaginable. Most of these cases are way too complex for the solo practitioner; if the patient in these scenarios took an interest in acupuncture, they would probably get it at a hospital under the auspices of an East–West program. However, it is instructive to read of these patients and see how they are treated.

Amber Walker is a PT who has first-hand experience with MCAS and hEDS. Her self-published book, *Mast Cells United: A Holistic Approach to Mast Cell Activation Syndrome* (2019), is itself a weighty volume. Her own health history, which she outlines in detail, is as astonishing as any that Dr. Afrin outlines. She is an exemplar of a certain subset of patient, and by this, I mean the ones who are so desperate for answers that they make researching their condition a second part-time job if not their sole full-time occupation. Social media groups provide mutual support and exchange of information, and to their credit, these suffering people do their research. Some, like Walker, write useful books. Her bibliography is exceptional and her explanation, in chapter two, of the different mast cells and what they do is a treasure. I always suggest to my MCAS patients that they read chapter two of *Mast Cells United*.

Neil Nathan's *Toxic: Heal Your Body from Mold Toxicity, Lyme Disease, Multiple Chemical Sensitivities, and Chronic Environmental*

*Illness* (2018) is a companion piece to the above two texts. Nathan is an MD in Vermont and this book reads like it was written by someone's crunchy uncle who also happens to be a doctor. He outlines differences between inflammation and toxicity and provides healthy guidelines for resolving each scenario. MCAS, Lyme disease, and mold toxicity are complex and potentially profoundly disabling issues but there are options. These three books, read one after the other, in comparison with one another, speak volumes. Patients who come to us for a holistic approach will either have already read (and probably nearly even memorized) *Heal Your Body*; patients who have not yet read it are deeply grateful when we suggest it.

The biomedical framework and approach we see in Afrin, Walker, and Nathan gives us a well-rounded perspective on how patients, especially patients new to Chinese medicine, articulate their experiences with chronic illness. Developing this level of awareness helps us to understand our patients better and it helps us to couch our discourse in languages that they can comprehend. But what of our own perspectives, practices, and languages? We of course have our own discourses related to Wind, Heat, and Damp and their attack on channels and organs.

A TCM approach to constant, unrelenting inflammation is available via Dr. Li Xiu-Min, a faculty member and researcher at the Icahn School of Medicine at Mount Sinai. Dr. Li's book, *Traditional Chinese Medicine, Western Science, and the Fight Against Allergic Disease* (2016), outlines her work with children who are dangerously allergic to just about everything. Parents who are desperate seek out Dr. Li and she maintains a Facebook group for families.[10] Children who are covered with weeping sores and crusty scabs have parents who will try Chinese medicine and be grateful for it once they have exhausted all other avenues. Chinese medicine is not second best or alternative for these families. It is their only hope. Any of Dr. Li's three books are worth reading, but the one I mention here offers a fine outline of how this particular practitioner uses Chinese medicine to change the course of people's lives.

*TCM Case Studies: Autoimmune Disease* (Zeng, Fratkin and Wang 2014) read alongside *Fight Against Allergic Disease* builds a practitioner's knowledge base exponentially. Though there is a difference between CTD and HCTD, many of the syndrome pattern identifications overlap and, even better, we gain practice at setting forth our treatment principles and methods by following this and other useful case study texts.[11]

In conjunction with the books that I mention in this section is another fundamental volume. *Fluid Physiology and Pathology in Traditional Chinese Medicine* (Clavey 2020), like *Rheumatology*, is another dense text that requires multiple readings to fully unearth its wisdom. However, if we wish to treat MCAS and any version of histamine intolerance, we need to imbibe the knowledge that this particular book confers. There are not two or three main points to consider when we address the issue of MCAS. Afrin's book, with its relentless string of case studies that will boggle the mind, describes MCAS better than anyone can in a summary. What I can say, as a sufferer of this condition and as a practitioner who treats it, is that any attempt to resolve or ameliorate MCAS or histamine intolerance requires patience, consistency, flexibility, and thorough knowledge of multiple ways to read it and address it.

Working with protean conditions like these requires a vast knowledge base, and the books that I have suggested here are the bare minimum of what a practitioner must read before beginning.

## Earth School

Reading the *Pi Wei Lun* many times over provides a multi-pronged benefit. In terms of building cultural competence, we may notice how gratifying it is to read other translations that mention Li Dong-Yuan and his influence. Dr. Xuē, as he treated bodies in pain, relied on the wisdom of Dr. Li. Qin Bo-Wei, a noted physician of just one generation ago, refers to his predecessor in a translation accessible to English speakers. When we read with an eye for intertextual exchange, it helps us to mentally build a coherent big picture. Famous names of Chinese medicine exist outside of their own books. These names become more familiar. As we become more familiar with the source text, we go back to tertiary ones and understand that much more. Repeated reading of the *Pi Wei Lun* draws us closer to culture and history and language.

It is also an invaluable resource for the treatment of ailments rooted in the middle Jiao, as we know. And, as in the matter of MCAS and chronic inflammation, we start with the gut and we can resolve a number of dysfunctions in so doing. Set next to another translation, the *Extra Treatises Based on Investigation and Inquiry: A Translation of Zhu Dan-xi's Ge Zhi Yu Lun* (Yang 2004), we once again are able to construct and reconstruct meaning surrounding Chinese medicine both at its source and in its contemporary iteration.[12] Of course, practitioners are already reading these seminal works. My invitation in this context is to read them once again through the lens of HCTD and MCAS. Centering Zhu Dan-xi alongside Li Dong-Yuan, going back and forth and back and forth again, and filtering the fruit of our studies through the lens of wishing to be of genuine service to our complex illness patients will garner successes that we would never have achieved otherwise.[13]

My teacher reminded me in a recent conversation of the value of rereading the classics upon which we form our professional identities. "When you go back months later and read again," he said, "you are able to see with new eyes, and maybe you see something new this time." Li Dong-Yuan wrote during a period of great suffering caused by war, epidemic, and social upheaval. Are we now not in a similar situation? If it has been a while since the last reading of *Pi Wei Lun*, now more than ever is a great time to go back to this gem and to read his colleague's work alongside it.

Our patients, on the other hand, will not be quite as enchanted as we are by the work of our medical forebears. Instead, they will come to us shaped by popular culture, layperson-friendly accounts of healthy eating, and perceptions created by their surroundings. What, then, is accessible to our patients? How do they learn to navigate the vagaries of their own digestive processes and outcomes? And, most important of all, how can we be sure that we are speaking their language when we discuss matters of gut health with them?

Each practitioner will have their own interests and, of course, we will also need to work within our local scope-of-practice laws. However, if a person is so inclined, it can be useful to follow the development of nutrition trends. I'm not necessarily enthralled by popular-culture food-as-medicine narratives, but being aware of the latest findings regarding a keto diet or the choice to cut out entire food groups in the pursuit of gut health (plus thinness, inner peace, and transcendence) helps us to know what ideas currently shape our patients' nutritional zeitgeist. I also am a member of several social media groups that revolve around nutrition for MCAS or histamine intolerance or EDS in all its subtypes. Doing so helps me to learn about these topics and it also gives me the opportunity to take part in conversations with real people who are living with complex dietary situations. When I speak to patients in my office, I speak their language.

Practitioners will enjoy *Gut Feelings: The Microbiome and Our Health* (Fasano and Flaherty 2021). Reading this, replete with the latest findings on the gut microbiome, we can feel extremely proud of Li Dong-Yuan who was so ahead of his time. If we need our predecessor's ideas translated into modern language that expresses through the constructs of gut bacteria, this is an enjoyable and pleasant way to make that connection. What does current science say, in clear terms, about gut bacteria? Fasano is a tenured professor at Harvard and Flaherty is the director of his health center there. The narrative contained within this popular-press rendering is the public-facing version of what is being studied in his laboratories and taught to his students. How does it align with what we know? In what way does it correspond with what Li Dong-Yuan and Zhu Dan-xi had to say?

I am disinclined to suggest a reading list for nutritional trends other than *Gut Feelings*, mainly because there is a vast wealth of material and it is beyond the scope of *Chinese Medicine* to delve into the vagaries of popular narrative surrounding food and diet. However, *A Silent Fire: The Story of Inflammation, Diet and Disease* (2022) by transplant gastroenterologist and assistant professor of medicine at Columbia University Medical Center, Shilpa Ravella, is worth mentioning. She begins by relating the start of her best friend's descent into life-threatening mystery illness. What follows, interspersed with returns to this friend's puzzling condition, is a history that encompasses everything from food to germs to environmental illness and more. Not everyone knows that the first fecal transplant, then called "yellow soup," took place in China in the fourth century under the direction of medical practitioner He Gong, but yes, she gives credit where credit is due. Chronic inflammation is a pressing topic in contemporary culture, and an enjoyable, substantive, and fast-paced survey of it can be found in Ravella's book.[14]

These texts, when read together, invoke a culture and language. Reading them, we gain a clearer understanding of our patients. We also gain useful information about how both Western biomedicine and popular culture frame and address these conditions. We may then gratefully return to Li Dong-Yuan and Zhu Dan-xi and take quite a bit of pride in how much they knew even without the structure provided by modern scientific narrative. We see the value of these and other similar texts when we keep in mind, as we should at all times, that culture counts.

Which brings me to the final entries for our comparative readings.

## Culture and Context

It is with great restraint that I refrain from going off on tangents about the role of the sick or weak body (or mind) in literature and art. I will not digress into an interrogation of the object of gazes or how women's bodies and those of marginalized groups function as lightning rods for social anxiety or leverage for hegemonic forces. This is not a literature class. And yet...and yet. We cannot begin to work with chronic illness and disability without reviewing how the recipients of our healthcare practice move within a larger system that can disempower them in ways that we might not even imagine unless we step back and view from a broad perspective.

*Doing Harm: The Truth About How Bad Medicine and Lazy Science Leave Women Dismissed, Misdiagnosed, and Sick* (2019) is thorough, compelling, and damning. In it, journalist Maya Dusenbery outlines a history of women's roles in the development of the biomedical industrial complex. It should be required reading for anyone in medicine, Western or Chinese. For those of us who treat chronic illness patients, especially ones who have been gaslit, it is a sine qua non. Some of our patients must navigate the corridors of Western biomedicine whether or not they want to do so; reading this book helps us to become better advocates. Other patients do not need to work with a biomedical doctor but we still can understand them better and help them more effectively if we understand the root causes of their mistrust. *Doing Harm* is meticulously sourced and compelling. We cannot meaningfully treat chronic illness, especially chronic illness in our female-identifying patients, without reading this book.

Two popular-press memoirs of chronic illness bring to life the themes outlined in *Doing Harm*. These are *The Lady's Handbook for her Mysterious Illness* (Ramey 2020) and *The Invisible Kingdom: Reimagining Chronic Illness* (O'Rourke 2022). Illness memoirs of course are a genre and there are many worthy candidates for inclusion in our interdisciplinary project, but the latter details the plight of a woman with hEDS and includes a relevant laundry list of adjacent conditions. If we wish to understand how the scenarios depicted in *Doing Harm* play out for a person with an HCTD, then *The Invisible Kingdom* is required reading. I have sprinkled quotes from *The Invisible Kingdom* throughout this book for a reason. O'Rourke almost ignores her EDS diagnosis in her memoir, which of course drew my attention, but her depiction of how she experienced mystery chronic illness sparkles with life and emotion. She invites readers to understand what it means to fear not being seen or understood. In my estimation and based on my clinical experience, the themes that O'Rourke illuminates in her memoir are ones that we, should we aspire to meaningful treatment of mystery disease, all need to know well.

In *The Lady's Handbook*, a reader will follow the contours of complex mystery illness that takes a detour into Chinese medicine and other "alternative" therapies in the translocal way that Mei Zhan describes in *Other-Worldly: Making Chinese Medicine through Transnational Frames* (2009). Herein, the author is a desperate patient who will try just about anything in order to find relief.[15] Without question, we view such patients with compassion and understanding, but we also remain aware of how their narratives may or may not shape public perception of Chinese medicine.

Whether or not such patients help or hurt themselves (and us) when consuming Chinese medicine this way is another book in and of itself. The value of this book lies elsewhere. *The Lady's Handbook* is a well-written, engaging, worthy memoir. Its author was an undergraduate when, suddenly, she developed one illness that led to another which led to a cascade of pain and disability and, to add insult to injury, her problems centered in her vagina. She endured excruciating pain. I had a good idea of what happened by about halfway into the narrative but that is only because I deal with chronic-illness mystery patients. And sure enough...well. I will leave it to readers of *Chinese Medicine* to read this book. We can notice how acupuncture fits into the larger picture herein (it does not shine a flattering light on the profession, though to be fair we only have the author's side of the story, not the acupuncturist's). We will gasp in horror at the depiction of the yoga instructor who shoves down on Ramey's hips and tells her to breathe through her pain. We will also notice how, in the conclusion, Ramey shares a letter from her doctor father and how she seems validated by his approval of her healthcare choices.

How we might react to particular aspects of *The Lady's Handbook* (and I think it is clear that I have my reservations regarding it), this is a book that merits reading. Working with patients with mystery illnesses requires compassion for those who lurch from naturopath to functional medicine doctor to acupuncturist and back again. They are part of a larger cultural fabric that is described very, very well by Ms. Ramey. If we are to treat patients like this with any integrity whatsoever, we need to read both the scientific accounts (Afrin, especially) and the social (Ramey, O'Rourke, Dusenbery) narratives. There is more to treatment of disease than syndromes or patterns or genetics and standards of care and scope-of-practice laws. Especially when the condition is so very complicated, we will always wish to step back and view, with knowledgeable eyes, the bigger pictures.

And yet, and especially when we may notice that Chinese medicine may seem devalued, or only valuable as a second choice, we must, as well, have resources that encourage us.

For me, the book that holds an honored place next to *Applied Channel Theory* is Liu Lihong's *Classical Chinese Medicine* (2019). This is a book that will help us to learn to think. There is also a continuous thread of defense for Chinese medicine and an unyielding refusal to accept any sense of second-class status for it. Read alongside Karchmer's excellent *Prescriptions for Virtuosity: The Postcolonial Struggle of Chinese Medicine* (2022), we are reminded of the efforts in certain sectors to defend the validity of this medicine. As the profession as a whole develops closer ties with evidence-based medicine and laboratory research, we always remember that this is a medicine that does have its own terms and this is a tradition that has had to fight for survival.

Will we do our part to keep it alive?

My choice for our interdisciplinary reading list in this realm oscillates. Some days, I review Mei Zhan's *Other-Worldly: Making Chinese Medicine through Transnational Frames* because it clarifies the way Chinese medicine was brought to the United States and repackaged. If we are not Asian American or of Asian heritage, we benefit from learning what Asian scholars who live their own version of being far from Beijing have to say.[16] This book is a good one to read either before or after Karchmer's field study and it, too, presents a cogent argument for a postcolonialist lens. And yet, my constant companion in daily work remains Deadman *et al.*'s *A Manual of Acupuncture* (2007). It sparks my joy to continue learning about points and their histories, their indications, and their cautions. Read next to *Classical Chinese Medicine*, I feel myself growing ever closer to understanding what to me is an authentic practice capable of adequately serving a complex patient population.

Another scholar's experience will be different than mine, but we mindfully read, and we meaningfully learn, when we compare and search for relations, not givens.


## III. ¿Crisol? o ¿Ensalada Mixta?

Over the course of my academic career, I have taught at institutions where the majority of the class was of Spanish-speaking heritage (University of New Mexico, Central New Mexico Community College, albeit Technical Vocational Institute (TVI) when I taught there) and at schools (I won't name names) where I was an exotic representative of Spain and southern Italy for most of the students. There is a middle ground, and I have taught in those institutions as well. In other words, in any given classroom there was a percentage of students with varying levels of connection to Spanish- or Italian-speaking cultures and communities and others with little to no experience in these realms. It is always interesting to ask the students if we, in the United States, are a melting pot or a mixed salad. The former is a trope that most know, and the responses varied. Some students I have asked genuinely felt that American identity meant speaking English as "our" official language and that fitting in and letting go of the practices of one's native culture is an admirable goal. Others vehemently opposed the notion of fitting in at the cost of one's cultural identification.

Popularized especially following the production of a play of the same name in 1908, the melting pot metaphor of a blend of ethnicities into one—an American, monocultural one—appealed to the zeitgeist of that time. In the 1960s, the notion that different groups could co-exist, each maintaining their cultural markings, gave rise to the idea of a salad bowl. Rather than melting into one homogenous whole, social groups can be comprised of varying parts that are mixed and in close quarters but which retain their boundaries. We recollect that this time frame—roughly 1910 through the 1960s—encompassed a period of intense debate in China regarding the value of Chinese medicine in the face of an ever-encroaching biomedical incursion. Whether or not one must give up one's identity in order to fit in and become part of an integrated (or hegemonic, depending on one's perspective) structure was not just an issue for immigrants to the United States of America during this period.

In what way might we consider the idea of a mixed salad vs. a melting pot with respect to the development of medical history, both within China and across the globe?[17]

If I were teaching a class on the cultural history of Chinese medicine, I would ask the students to debate the question of whether, as practitioners of Chinese medicine outside of China, we are mung bean paste tucked into mooncakes or we are ingredients in a communal hot pot. Are we congee or are we bags of rice? Often, when teaching people to step out of their normal, it is more effective and fun to do it in a way that makes people laugh.

Another approach is to encourage conversation about something other, something that is non-threatening and then, when students are accustomed to the topic, to bring it close to home. I used to do this with conversations about the American Southwest and our border states. Italy and Spain are relatively small countries whose imperialism left scars on their southern neighbors. Now, when the influx of desperately poor Africans and Latin Americans is cause for hostility and debate, it is worth asking whose responsibility this is, and it is worth considering how much Spain and Italy owe their neighbors now. Students could really get into that conversation, and when they did, I'd at some point or another ask them to turn the focus towards the United States and our neighbors to the south. Students who might have gotten extremely upset by this topic if I had started with the United States were able to cope with it because they were already engaged with the broader picture via a focus on a non-threatening other country, one not theirs.

I wonder, then, how we might broach similar conversations within the profession as it is developing outside of China and independent, now, of its point of origin. How might a practitioner, when faced with illnesses that do not necessarily have easy answers in either an Eastern or a Western medical approach, parse through the options and ultimately provide the safest, healthiest, and most efficacious treatment? How do we filter Chinese medicine through our language, culture, and legal boundaries regarding scope of practice? Ultimately, are we mung bean paste or are we hot pot? What, in effect, are the ingredients that make a practitioner and what, with these ingredients, is produced and consumed?

We have much to offer and we can, in fact, provide considerable benefit to patients with Chinese tradition rather than via bowdlerized medicine that is so integrated that it no longer shares even a family resemblance to its originator. Patients desperately need what we can bring to the table and we do not, in order to bring it, need to lose contact with the heart of Chinese medicine. The Ehlers-Danlos syndromes are complex and variable but they can be alleviated if one opts for one of the four areas that I have outlined in this book: Bi syndrome, the Earth School, via nurturing of the shen, or by reconsidering notions surrounding Gu syndrome. One of the gifts of treating HCTDs is that this specialty invites a practitioner to continue studying, and to study widely.

There is something for everyone in this hot pot of Chinese medical tradition. What matters is that we find our threads and follow them, confidently, and with a wide base of knowledge.

# Conclusion

"Chinese medicine is as dear to me as my own skin" (2019, p.3) declares Liu Lihong. This is the first sentence of *Classical Chinese Medicine* and it is as much an affirmation as it is a direct challenge to the reader. Leaving aside the literal value of this organ—the largest organ of our body—we may consider its metaphorical worth. What does this protective barrier and thermal regulator mean to each one of us? We may not take note of it unless, perhaps, it turns against us with faulty collagen or when the cutaneous nerves attack via agonizing small fiber neuropathy. It could be that we are fortunate and able to love our skin. That he cherishes this medicine as much as he does that which encompasses him from top to toe, his skin, is a call to action for anyone who sees these words. Dr. Liu wants us, his readers, to know the value of this medicine. Though his arguments come back again and again in favor of reading the classics, he also brings concepts surrounding the clinical encounter to the forefront. Over the course of his book, he illuminates our path to Beijing, adding that, "In particular, I hope that this discourse provides the reader with a sound foundation for a correct understanding of Chinese medicine" (*ibid.*, p.3).

There is not one way to diagnose or treat any complex illness and I know that I am not alone when I say that Chinese medicine is as dear to me as my own skin too. The world over, practitioners and patients alike whose lives have been changed by this form of healing will express the same sentiment and know, to their very bones, that it is true.

Chinese medicine is excellent medicine and it is particularly apt for the chronic diseases that are becoming so common. That does not mean to say that it is medicine of last resort to be sampled when everything else has failed and nothing seems to work. No. Chinese medicine is excellent medicine for the kinds of complex illnesses that we are seeing today. We as a profession, no matter where we practice, are already prepared to respond to a growing need for our services. As O'Rourke notes in *The Invisible Kingdom: Reimagining Chronic Illness*, "Today, to treat the growing numbers of patients living with these amorphous, system-roaming illnesses, medicine may need to return to a model of disease at the core of ancient medicine, one that sees sickness as a disruption of a particular body's natural balance" (2022, pp.43–44). She's right. The line drawing of the human figure with a whole world within it that we see in our Chinese medicine textbooks is entirely apt for this moment within which we find ourselves today. We are part of a microcosm and our larger environment today is battered by a myriad of forces. I doubt that anyone could convincingly argue otherwise.

Chinese medicine is valuable medicine, and in this cultural moment that is wrought by climate change, social upheaval, pandemic, and ever-increasing rare and complex disease, we might even say that its moment has arrived. Western biomedicine does not have all the answers. Nobody does. We do have a lot to say from our own patch of earth, though.

But—and this is a big one—we are tasked with not only helping patients but also finding our identities as practitioners. Dr. Liu, like other sources I discussed throughout *Chinese Medicine*, expresses concern about how current and future practitioners will learn, stating that, "We must consider whether this personalized [i.e., lineage-based] teaching is possible without the essential one-on-one mentorship of the traditional model" (2019, p.40). He laments that, "The old masters are gradually passing from this world, and their successors are university graduates who have no experience and sense of true teacher–disciple transmission and therefore do not know how to find and teach suitable disciples themselves" (*ibid.*, p.41). People in China who are fortunate enough to have access to classical scholarship have their own barriers to learning and those of us in far-flung lands must walk our own paths.

What, then, to do?

It is for this reason that I argue for the thought processes and scholarly practices of comparative literature and cultural studies. This is why I argue for a wide range of readings beyond those assigned in our programs for Chinese or integrative medicine. In the introduction to *Comparative Literature in an Age of Globalization* (2006), Haun Saussy might sound pretentious when he states that, "Comparative literature is best known, not as the reading *of literature*, but as reading *literarily* (with intensive textual scrutiny, defiance, and metatheoretical awareness) whatever there may be to read" (p.23), but what can I say, other than to offer up the colloquial rejoinder, "No lies detected"? Furthermore, as he states, "we are good at interdisciplinarity, which is easy to do badly" (*ibid.*, p.34). Dr. Liu argues for reading the Chinese medical classics, noting that, "Serious study of the classics is able to stretch the limits of our understanding, to broaden our perspective" (2019, p.55) and he is correct. But, and especially if we are foreign to this tradition, it is not altogether that easy to grasp the soul of these readings.

Even if we do read classical Chinese, even if we are actually a native Chinese person from a venerable scholar-physician family, we still have a lot of learning to do before we can truly comprehend the texts and apply their wisdom to living patients sitting before us. When we treat HCTDs and other extremely complicated disorders, we lift our noses from our books and look at the patient who comes to us with their own story and their own narrative and must ask ourselves the eternal question: *and what else?* In the absence of a diagnosis, we are required to fill in the blanks of their stories. That takes a lot of extra reading, no matter one's subject position or ease with the native language and culture.

Hence this book, in so many ways.

O'Rourke is especially apt, once again, as a supporting voice to my arguments here. I practice in the United States, but clinicians in other countries will have their own thoughts on the matter of humility and the need to be able to say, "I don't know." These three small words can do so much more than we might think to reassure our patients. That sense of not feeling seen, she explains, went beyond the lack of diagnosis, "Rather, I had felt invisible in my illness, I realized, because American culture—and American medicine within it—largely strives to downplay the fact that we still know so little about illness. A doctor friend told me that in med school he was explicitly taught never to say 'I don't know' to a patient. Uncertainty was thought to open the door to lawsuits" (2022, p.130). Western medicine is uncomfortable with nuance and uncertainty; Chinese medicine, within its own environs and teachings, is not.

But we do labor against certain pernicious forms of received wisdom when we step out of our own professional milieux. I remember once, while I was early in my program, going to get the oil in my car changed. While the service was in progress, I was sitting on a bench by the door to the repair bay and studying for—if memory serves me correctly—one of my point location exams. My eyes were closed and I was trying to memorize, and when the mechanic came to tell me that my car was ready, I jumped at the sound of his voice. He apologized, and when I said that I was reviewing for an exam, he replied that he had thought I was praying. I laughed and said, "Well, I probably should be, but anyhow..." We had a chat about Chinese medicine, then, and he told me that his wife had died of breast cancer. This was recent, he said. He told me that she loved acupuncture and that she had gotten a lot of it after her mastectomy and chemo. "It didn't work though," he told me, "She died anyway."

I wanted to say to him that Chinese medicine did not fail his wife. The mastectomy and the chemotherapy "didn't work" and the acupuncture probably made her a lot more comfortable in the process. It "worked" very well for its purpose, which is probably why she loved it and got a lot of it in her final months. But I couldn't say this to the poor old man as he stood in front of me with his eyes shining and full of sudden tears. Instead, I gave him a hug and told him that I was sorry for his loss.

When Western medicine does not know or makes a mistake, received wisdom holds that it is a matter of not having data and finally acquiring enough data. It is not that it's bad medicine or lacking in some way. Conversely, when Chinese medicine doesn't know, we must defend ourselves against the perception that it's because we're not as sophisticated or we don't have the modern technology. When it doesn't work, we need to push back against the idea that it's because it's not real medicine anyway or is somehow lacking (unless of course we have a heartbroken elderly widower standing in front of us, then, I think, one is forgiven for seeing only the sorrow and overlooking the erroneous thought process). To anyone who has not studied Chinese medicine, my answer to charges that we are primitive or lacking comes from Dr. Liu: "If you have yet to truly understand Chinese medicine theory, or at the very least to have attained what resembles an understanding of Chinese medicine theory, what basis do you have to determine whether it is primitive or advanced?" (2019, p.7). But to my professional peers, I would also say that we need to be comfortable saying that we do not know.

It is a mixture of yin and yang, really, only in this context I am referring to being both confident and humble. "I do not know" can balance with "but I can find out." Western biomedicine is coming to the conclusion that this is a valuable skill, too. According to David Putrino, director of rehabilitation innovation for the Mount Sinai Health System and long COVID expert, "'A lot of clinicians want the algorithm'… 'There is no algorithm. There is listening to your patient, identifying symptoms, finding a way to measure the severity of the symptoms, applying interventions to them, and then seeing if those symptoms resolve. That is the way medicine should be'" (quoted in O'Rourke 2022, p.255). If we ponder it, this is the way Chinese medicine is already, and I think we already know that this is so. We only need, I think, to reinforce our confidence in this medicine *as it is* and without undue reliance on validation from biomedicine. We need to recognize that both medical traditions, Asian and Western, would do better by approaching chronic complex illness with the balance of I do not know and I can find out (or at least: I am willing to try to find out).

Arthur Frank, in *The Wounded Storyteller: Bodies, Illness, and Ethics* (2013), outlines three types of illness stories, categorizing them as either restitution narratives, chaos narratives, or quest narratives. In the first, getting better is the story. Things get resolved. In the second, it's one mess after the next and nothing really gets fixed. In the third, the person is ennobled by synthesis and the discovery of meaning in the illness. Of these three options, O'Rourke relates that, "The more I talked to sick people, the more I found that what is most disturbing for many of us is that grace has become a kind of moral requirement in sickness: *If you must be ill, at least be* improved *by your illness*" (2022, p.261). I do not think it's up to the patient to be improved by their illness, though. I think it is up to us, the practitioners, to become improved in their stead.

Dr. Liu would remind that, and I quote, "The ancients said: 'Read a book a hundred times and its meaning will be self-evident'" (2019, p.76). The question, then, is: which books? We need to know what we do not know for patient safety (Western medicine needs to do the same) and so we read our Chinese medicine textbooks and compare them against the biomedicine ones. We also need to know what we do not know for the sake of the patient's own sense of selfhood, and for that, we read from history and anthropology and literature. We look at works of art and ask ourselves about their creation. We learn to trace narrative threads the way we become adept at outlining syndromes and patterns. In so doing, we learn to look, and we learn to see.

Above all, we must always, *always* come back around to the patient and their experience with their complex disorder. The current and pressing focus on finding a specific gene for hEDS is understandable but there are multiple strands to this thread. Is hEDS rooted in MCAS, as Dr. Afrin posits? I think for some of us, it is. I know that when I read Afrin's article, my response was to tear up a little bit and think: *I FEEL SEEN*. (We all want to feel seen.) For some, the argument that hEDS is a manifestation of autism is persuasive. A person with an identified alteration in the MTHFR gene leading to impaired processing of B vitamins may find recourse in specific supplements to address that lack and thus, ultimately, find relief from their hEDS presentation. A genetic mutation, if ever identified, might not change their story much, if at all. Patients with complex disorders will still need to develop their narrative surrounding them and practitioners are able to provide the very best care when we are able to hear them, to listen, and to truly see.

I began this conclusion with a quote from Dr. Liu and I will end with another. In pondering the question of motivation, he sternly tells us to, "Ask yourself, therefore, the question of how you came to this profession" (*ibid.*, p.48). What brought us here, which road we take to get to Beijing, what we will do once there... these are all individualized questions with unique answers from all of us.

Where, now, does your journey begin?

# Notes

## Chapter 1

1   The majority of the online resources I cite throughout *Chinese Medicine* are current or relatively recent and this is for a reason: interest in hypermobility is increasing exponentially the world over. A study of generalized joint hypermobility (GJH) in American university students showed a rate of 12.5% in survey participants (Reuter and Fichthorn, tinyurl.com/mr2xy3rp). Data analysis of electronic health records in Wales by Demmler *et al.* revealed that roughly 15–20% of the population is hypermobile; in consequence, they argue that classifying hEDS and hypermobility spectrum disorders as rare merits reconsideration (tinyurl.com/4d28pbx9).

2   Diagnosis and diagnostics represent a recurring theme in any discussion of EDS and constitute a pervasive topic in this book. Noted researcher, Lawrence Afrin, lamented the absence of genetic markers for hEDS in his 2021 article "Some cases of hypermobile Ehlers-Danlos syndrome may be rooted in mast cell activation syndrome," while private donations support what is known as the HEDGE (Hypermobile Ehlers-Danlos Genetic Evaluation) study that is currently underway (tinyurl.com/t2tn3zbc). Changes in categorization have meant that people who would have been diagnosed under older criteria are now not eligible for diagnosis, which alarms those who do want this confirmation. There is both a patient-safety element to diagnosis and a cultural aspect to the question of identifying as being a person with hEDS, among many other facets of this theme. Though research findings in 2021 point to a forthcoming official identification of an aberrant gene associated with hEDS, issues surrounding the question of diagnosis will not be going anywhere at any time soon. Understanding its parameters is key to understanding the Ehlers-Danlos syndromes.

3   At Warwick University in England, Sabeeha Malek is undertaking research that focuses on aberrations in cell adhesion and cytoskeleton dynamics; according to her theory, the extracellular matrix (ECM) has a substantive involvement in tissue dysfunction. Refer to "The role of cell adhesion and cytoskeleton dynamics in the pathogenesis of the Ehlers-Danlos syndromes and hypermobility spectrum disorders" (Malek and Köster, tinyurl.com/5n6seh4a).

4    The fourteenth subtype was discovered in 2018 and thus is not yet included in the official categorization of EDS set forth at the 2017 International Consortium on the Ehlers-Danlos Syndromes. The Ehlers-Danlos Society online reports that there are only four individuals from three different families with the newly identified genetic defect ("A new type of Ehlers-Danlos syndrome discovered" tinyurl.com/56bn3s6j).

5    There are a number of online resources addressing knowledge of and comfort levels with hEDS, both in popular accounts and in research studies. This is not only a matter of patients wanting support or guidance; practitioners are also uncertain and in need of useful information. Because EDS is of global concern, I share here a sample from Scotland (Dockrell, Berg and Ralston, "Mind the gaps: Therapists' experiences of managing symptomatic hypermobility in Scotland" tinyurl.com/3auma6m5), the United States (Jones and Black, "Provider knowledge and experience in care, management, and education of pediatric Ehlers-Danlos syndrome" tinyurl.com/bdfn92c2), and Italy (Sulli *et al.*, "Ehlers-Danlos syndromes: State of the art on clinical practice guidelines" tinyurl.com/44wnbv2k). It is worth noting that I wrote two blog posts in 2017 and 2018, respectively, and have subsequently been contacted with requests for information about Chinese medicine's treatment of EDS from practitioners in Spain, France, Belgium, England, Canada, and multiple locations across the United States. These emailed queries were the inspiration for this book.

6    Unless otherwise specified, general information regarding EDS is sourced from The Ehlers-Danlos Society (www.ehlers-danlos.com), Ehlers-Danlos Support UK (www.ehlers-danlos.org), or the National Organization for Rare Disorders (https://rarediseases.org).

7    "The trifecta" as a collection does not always meet with agreement. A relatively recent article by Kohn and Chang, "The relationship between hypermobile Ehlers-Danlos Syndrome (hEDS), postural orthostatic tachycardia syndrome (POTS), and mast cell activation syndrome (MCAS)" (tinyurl.com/2p83eujk), argues for a lack of evidence of this connection. PT Amber Walker's 2021 book, *The Trifecta Passport: Tools for Mast Cell Activation Syndrome, Postural Orthostatic Tachycardia Syndrome and Ehlers-Danlos Syndrome*, stringently advocates otherwise. Chronic illness communities are adamantly supportive of Walker's position. Noted researcher, physician, and MCAD/MCAS authority Lawrence Afrin theorizes, as mentioned above in note 2, that MCAS may be directly related to hEDS.

8    There are three different types of POTS: neuropathic, whereby the sympathetic nerves do not properly stimulate vessels, thus impeding blood flow from lower limbs; hyperadrenergic, which is when the patient has a high level of norepinephrine in their blood, which generally leads to high blood pressure and the heightened heart rate; and secondary POTS, which is tachycardia upon changing position due to other causes, like diabetes or

lupus or alcoholism. In my experience, the hEDS patients I have seen with POTS have had the first type.

9   Similar to the trifecta, MCAS presents controversy in some quarters. Valent and Akin's article, "Doctor, I think I am suffering from MCAS: Differential diagnosis and separating facts from fiction" (tinyurl.com/25eh8hj3), was met with genuine outrage in online communities. That MCAS exists is not questionable; the issue, instead, is whether or not a patient can get a diagnosis or if they are told by their doctor that they are hypersensitive and overly imaginative.

10  The distinction between histamine intolerance and MCAS is a fine one. Interpretations of it are, in part, predicated on location, as Cimolai notes, "Overall, the clinical presentation of HI [histamine intolerance] is generally confusing. It is of note that much of the published literature on this topic arises from central Europe. The clinical symptomatology of HI, although diverse and hence confusing, has a remarkable similarity to non-clonal mast cell activation syndrome (NC-MCAS) which is gathering increasing attention, but especially in North America" (tinyurl.com/4nm9xe8a).

11  Though practitioners are not likely to see patients with this condition in our clinics, we would, should we have EDS patients, wish to be aware that headache, high blood pressure, or pulsatile tinnitus in this population might warrant extra consideration and a referral to their PCP. One resource for further information is the NORD's link, accessible here: tinyurl.com/54w9rsx2, that discusses FMD in the context of vEDS and Marfan syndrome, among other predispositions, while a 2020 study written up by Otman announced a newly discovered genetic variant associated with cEDS ("Genetic study uncovers mutation associated with fibromuscular dysplasia" tinyurl.com/ysr7ksxa).

12  "Endocrine abnormalities in hereditary disorders of connective tissue" (McDonnell, tinyurl.com/bdew3u5r).

13  Rodgers *et al.* analyzed electronic health record data and published their findings in "Ehlers-Danlos syndrome hypermobility type is associated with rheumatic diseases" (tinyurl.com/yc4tcnnt).

14  Frigid extremities can also be caused by dysautonomia and this presentation can be quite serious, as Soloway *et al.* in "Cyanosis with dysautonomia mimics Raynaud disease" demonstrate (tinyurl.com/4mkbn4kw).

15  The plight of patients who are misdiagnosed with fibromyalgia is common knowledge in chronic illness communities. A global call for change by GERSED Belgique is "Fibromyalgia or Ehlers-Danlos syndrome(s)?" (tinyurl.com/44xtp2pf).

16  See Langhinrichsen-Rohling *et al.* "They've been BITTEN: Reports of institutional and provider betrayal and links with Ehlers-Danlos Syndrome patients' current symptoms, unmet needs and healthcare expectations" (tinyurl.com/mvsp39t4).

17  Noted researcher, physician, and expert on chronic illness, Dr. Michael D. Lockshin, writes in *The Prince at the Ruined Tower: Time, Uncertainty, and Chronic Illness* (hereafter *Prince*), "Doctors have two duties: To diagnose and to prescribe. From Hippocrates to Galen, from Ibn Sina to Maimonides, and up to this very day, symptoms and diagnosis, prescription and cure, that has been the rule" (2017, p.179). For its part, *Prince* offers a book-length discussion of the uncertainty and challenges inherent in working with chronic illness. Lockshin's specialty area is rheumatology in general and lupus in particular, and the entirety of *Prince* can be read as an investigation of the theme of diagnosis.

18  Marfan syndrome presents on a spectrum and there are people who embody Marfanoid traits but who do not fit within the diagnostic category per se. This is a challenge for clinicians to diagnose, as Wozniak-Mielcza-rek *et al.*'s "How to distinguish Marfan syndrome from Marfanoid Habitus in a physical examination—Comparison of external features in patients with Marfan Syndrome and Marfanoid Habitus" (tinyurl.com/4bb4kfyf) makes clear. As this article explains, a Marfan syndrome diagnosis is significant and not one to be given lightly. For the sake of patient safety, we need to be aware of this syndrome and its signs. Ultimately, we can be of tremendous service to patients when we are able to point them in the right direction towards appropriate biomedical intervention when there are red flags. A resource that I have found very useful in this regard is https://marfan.org.


# Chapter 2


1  A central theme in Karchmer's analysis of contemporary Chinese attitudes towards indigenous medicine revolves around efficacy and chronic vs. acute illness. In his introduction, Karchmer promises to, "examine the prejudice that Chinese medicine is only suitable for treating chronic illness, as expressed in the phrase that 'Western medicine treats acute illness; Chinese medicine treats chronic illness' (*xiyi zhi jixingbing; zhongyi zhi manxingbing*)" (2022, p.25). Like Karchmer, I find this attitude regrettable. Chinese medicine is exceptional for acute illness *and* I am very, very proud of what we can do for our chronic illness patients.

2  The relative weight given to disease-focused vs. syndrome-preferential diagnostic approaches is a sensitive issue. In *Chinese Medicine: Theories of Modern Practice Volume I*, Wiseman and Wilms's introduction avers that translated textbooks give the erroneous impression that Chinese medicine is not disease oriented. They point out that: "The present text has over 130 disease terms commonly appearing in Chinese-language basic theory textbooks. This radically changes Western perception of Chinese medicine

discussing mainly patterns rather than diseases" (2020, p.iv). In *Classical Chinese Medicine*, Liu Lihong firmly declares that, "to say that Chinese medicine does not differentiate between diseases and only analyzes the syndrome is a gross misunderstanding" (2019, p.175).

3   In *Prescriptions for Virtuosity*, Karchmer declares his intention early on, stating that, "I hope to bridge a concerning divide in the scholarship on Chinese medicine in which historical research has often been divorced from the contemporary concerns of clinical practice and ethnographic research mistakes recent innovations for timeless, ahistorical traditions" (2022, p.25). I think, in agreement with Karchmer, that we are quite overdue for an interrogation of some of the received wisdom proclaimed by ethnographic research.

4   Learning any new language, from Spanish to Chinese or any other, is challenging, and ancient versions are that much more difficult. Spanish is a standardized language but medieval Castilian is not easy to read, even for native speakers. I remember as an undergraduate in comparative literature struggling through excerpts of Chaucer in the original, and Old English texts like *Beowulf* gave me panic attacks. Dante's Tuscan, cleansed in the Arno as it may be, does not submit to language apps as does contemporary spoken Italian. However, I do think that Chinese medicine programs should require students to undertake at least a term or two of the language and I know that some at this time do.

5   In some ways, being of the community that one researches or treats or teaches can be a bonus. We enjoy a certain level of authenticity simply by being ourselves. It is also easier to understand when one has first-hand experience. Having a bone that routinely pops out of its socket might be hard to comprehend for someone who has never known the feeling. Empathizing with a patient as they describe how their lips swell and the roof of their mouth peels off when they eat anything but a few limited items is not hard, but to be able to know because one has experienced it is a completely different level of understanding. However, each presentation is so varied that a practitioner with hEDS might have a completely different experience than any of their HCTD patients. I thus caution against the equation of first-hand experience with clinical knowledge, even though it may be human nature to think this way. When I was a Spanish professor, for instance, I would occasionally have native speaker students from Spain or other countries. Every now and again, I would have a conflict with one or the other who felt that, because they were authentic specimens, they should be granted top grades simply for existing. My rejoinder was to say that if authenticity granted complete knowledge, then all American students should be given automatic A grades in their history and English composition classes because, after all, they are nationals and this is their native language. In sum: being a member of this population does not absolve any of us from doing all of our homework.

6    Taking recourse once again in Karchmer's scholarship, I found it encouraging to read how, according to his experience, contemporary Chinese doctors opt to, "First diagnose a disease, then determine a pattern (*xian bianbing, zai bianzheng*)," and that, "As this aphorism suggests, biomedicine predominates in the first stage of the diagnosis. But once this stage has been completed, doctors make a methodological shift from disease/*bing* diagnosis to *bianzheng lunzhi*. This shift creates a space in which doctors can practice Chinese medicine with greater freedom from the influence of Western medicine. This degree of freedom, however, depends to a large extent on the clinical skills of each individual physician" (2022, p.200). This is practical and, as per the concluding sentence, a reminder to all that we must become, absolutely and without question, the most skilled that we possibly can be.

7    There is a human element to the act of seeing that transcends diagnosis. Meghan O'Rourke, author of *The Invisible Kingdom*, says of her odyssey, "While there was no single answer, one thing stood out: above all, I wanted recognition of the reality of my experience, a sense that others saw it, not least because human ingenuity might then be applied to the disease that had undone me, so that others might in the future suffer less than I had" (2022, p.5).

8    Orthostatic hypotension can also be associated with hEDS and, like POTS, it causes dizziness, syncope, and other issues. With a "pretzel leg sign" the patient's legs will be twisted just as the name suggests. This is the body's effort to pump blood through the muscles in the lower limbs. This manifestation of autonomic nervous system dysfunction will often be accompanied by "coat hanger phenomenon," in which the shoulders and neck are painful in the shape of its name. As with the legs, pain is due to lack of blood flow throughout the muscles of the neck and shoulder. Goldstein's "Coat hanger phenomenon & the pretzel leg sign (14 of 24)" elucidates the clinical significance of these signs (tinyurl.com/4vnrj6hb). It is worth following the link in the article to Dr. Goldstein's YouTube channel because it is part 14 of an open-access online course titled "Introduction to Autonomic Medicine."

9    It helps us to know what the Beighton scale is but I do not use it as an assessment. I am also strongly disinclined to use range of motion (ROM) tests on patients with HCTDs. The risk of injuring a patient is high and someone with hEDS is usually going to have a remarkable range of motion even if they are, in the moment, stiff by their own standards. The Beighton is an assessment tool that gives a point for each side (right and left) being able to pull the little finger back past 90°, pull the thumb down all the way to the forearm, bend the elbows and/or knees back past 10°, and/or lie the hands flat on the floor while bending at the waist and maintaining straightened knees. The highest score is 9 and anything above a 5 is considered positive, although numbers change as a person ages. To

view the assessment via the Ehlers-Danlos Society, refer to tinyurl.com/ yc3nxc6d. For remarks on its validity, see "The Beighton Score as a measure of generalised joint hypermobility" (Malek, Reinhold and Pearce, tinyurl. com/2p9yvmdz). While valuable, the Beighton scale does have its detractors and its usefulness is akin to the way body mass index (BMI) is a tool that does not work for everyone.

10  A herd of zebras is called a dazzle and the hEDS community has happily adopted that term for its members.

11  My personal experience here is instructive. Before I developed MCAS as a result of pharmaceutical injury, I offered moxibustion treatments and found the odor of the herbs pleasant. I understood the idea that it might bother some patients. Once I experienced what it is like to live with MCAS and be overcome by the smell of moxibustion, however, I was genuinely shocked by how truly disparate the space between "understanding that it bothers some patients" vs. "being a person who had a hyper-reaction" is. My response to the scent of burning *Ai Ya* was that my upper lip swelled alarmingly, my throat tightened and I struggled to breathe comfortably, my heart pounded, I experienced a facial nerve pain flare so that I was in agony, and I literally felt like I was going to faint or drop dead. I managed to remain calm and remove myself from the trigger, but I share this anecdote with the invitation to colleagues in the profession to imagine what this would be like if one were a patient and new to Chinese medicine.

12  See also "The masseuse who pulled my arm out" (Clarke, tinyurl.com/ f9v35m8x). This story is shared in a humorous way and relates damage that was less severe than my patient's but, in both scenarios, the lesson regarding potential for injury is worth noting.

13  Allopathic physicians also find the initial intake to be challenging, as Bluestein's article "Shortening the diagnostic odyssey for hypermobile Ehlers-Danlos syndrome: A primer for the primary care physician" demonstrates (tinyurl.com/yckfezzf). Practitioners of Chinese medicine do not need to undergo the sort of elaborate process a biomedical clinic does in order to develop a practice in this area but Knight *et al.*'s description of the steps they had to undertake in order to do so in "Establishing an Ehlers-Danlos syndrome clinic: Lessons learned" is edifying. In conclusion, they note that, "Biomedical research has progressed as well to allow us to treat patients with the tools of medicine we have available. Unfortunately, there is often much that cannot yet be explained by biomedical knowledge, specifically pertaining to the link of illness and disease in patients with hEDS/HSD" and reiterate their commitment to a multidisciplinary practice (tinyurl.com/2s4eatf2).

14  Inokuchi *et al.* in "Vascular Ehlers-Danlos syndrome without the characteristic facial features: A case report" outline the, "large eyes, small chin, sunken cheeks, thin nose and lips, and lobeless ears" we might expect in a

vEDS patient (tinyurl.com/4wywkyje). The article is worth reading because it illuminates how challenging it is for biomedicine to diagnose patients and underscores how useful it can be when a Chinese medicine practitioner is knowledgeable. Though we are not the ones to diagnose, we can certainly be exceptionally good sources for education and awareness. We can also take note of signs and symptoms and help patients by identifying red flags.

15 Generally, patients who live with such extreme pain that they are given opioid drugs do not rely on Chinese medicine, and the author of the *Intractable Pain Patient's Handbook for Survival* specifically notes that the degree of pain his patients suffer is well beyond the capacity of acupuncture (Tennant 2021, p.1). This 93-page handbook is short and gives brutal, no-frills advice to those whose lives are entirely regulated by pain. It is worth reading even though its author is clearly not a fan of Chinese medicine. His presentation of survival tactics is sound, we learn quite a bit about what it means to live with extreme pain, and he has a section at the end with historical photographs and a brief biographical sketch of pain physicians and caretakers. Dr. Tennant is an interesting figure. He is mainly known for his work with adhesive arachnoiditis, an excruciatingly painful inflammation of the spinal canal. He was also an expert defense witness for Elvis Presley's doctor, who was accused of malpractice when the star died of an overdose. In *The Strange Medical Saga of Elvis Presley* (2021), Tennant hypothesizes that one of Presley's maladies was EDS.

16 Sabeeha Malek is a resource to follow for Chinese medicine practitioners who focus on maternal wellness. The EDS Maternity Co-Created Tools website to which she contributes may be useful for a specialist in hEDS and women's health (tinyurl.com/2p94j25j).

17 We readily speak of Stomach qi rebellion but lack a term for what happens when a person's wei qi revolts in the instance of MCAS. In my experience, my own ferocious and unstoppable wei qi has given me cause to refer to its activity as wei qi rebellion. Like the legendary inhabitants of Numancia in ancient Spain who decided that they would die before allowing themselves to be conquered by the Romans, a person with MCAS has wei qi that is willing to fight to the bitter end for its cause.

18 Dr. Liu's assertion, "The same disease is different to some degree in each person because each person's reaction to that disease is individual. This is called 'the same disease but a different syndrome.' The disease may be identical, but the syndrome might be altogether disparate" (2019, p.241), is a worthy reminder of received wisdom that we are assumed to already know. However, that he feels compelled to make this comment is telling. I think that we may begin to forget this precept as we become more and more familiar with our patient populations and treatment strategies. With HCTD patients, though, we take this admonition to heart.

19  Dr. Liu declares that, "There are at least four levels of ability among Chinese Medicine practitioners: the divine (*shen*), the sagely (*sheng*), the adept (*gong*), and the astute (*qiao*). To know by simply looking, this is divine; to listen and know is sagely; to ask and then to know is adept; to feel the pulse and know is astute"; either way, he concludes, "The syndromes of Chinese Medicine merit our best efforts to understand them" (2019, p.231).

20  Regarding the capacity to see an illness before it manifests, Dr. Liu also reminds us of the story of Zhang Zhongjing and the nobleman Wan Zhongxuan and how this venerable ancestor said, "Your highness has a disease. If not treated, your eyebrows will fall out at the age of 40, and then within a half a year, you will die" (2019, p.229). According to Dr. Liu, Zhang Zhongjing knew this because, "he discerned the syndrome (*zheng*)"; consequently, Dr. Liu instructs, this is evidence for the need to understand the syndrome, in that, "If you have a firm grasp of the syndrome, and you can peer into the essence of the rationale underlying that syndrome, then you can understand not only the disease that lies before you, but also those changes that it will undergo in the future" (p.230).

# Chapter 3

1  Not everyone wants to self-identify as disabled. Others take this identity as part of their very bones. We as practitioners can make the effort to comprehend a patient's identity and languages. Resources that support our learning include the Disability Language Style Guide page (https://ncdj.org/style-guide) from the American National Center on Disability and Journalism. Awareness of disability-inclusive language helps us not only to provide better care in our clinics. When we write our own blog posts or create our own marketing content, we can be attentive to how we frame our discourse. The entire website is instructive. They also link Spanish, Italian, and Romanian translations of their Guide, which of course made my Spanish professor's heart sing with joy.

2  "Medical acupuncture" is an interesting term. By now, it should be clear that I am extremely aware of language and the power of words. The first time I heard the term "medical acupuncture," I gasped out loud at the implications of it. If biomedical doctors perform "medical acupuncture," I thought, then what kind of acupuncture am I delivering? The kind that is unscientific, vaguely magical, and delivered by someone who is not medical and not working within a medical tradition? (The pejorative term "energy healer" sprang to mind.)

3  Each state in the USA has its own regulations for practitioners of Chinese medicine, and in California, New Mexico, and Florida, acupuncturists are PCPs. Each country has its own laws and it is instructive to see how these

laws are applied globally. For further information, see Calduch's "Regulation of Chinese medicine in the different countries of the world" (tinyurl.com/yckmtz3y).

4   Dr. Liu makes an excellent point and he couches it within his classical frame of reference. To wit: "Zhang Zhongjing sets forth from the three yin and the three yang. Li Dongyuan begins with the spleen and stomach. Ye Tianshi analyzes disease in terms of the four levels: defensive, qi, nutritive, and blood. Wu Jutong explains physiology and pathology in terms of the three burners. Following any of these methods to their final destination, we arrive at an accurate understanding: we 'arrive at Beijing.' All of these methods reveal the truth, the Dao" (2019, p.385). Chinese medicine is so rich and expansive. We must guard against going off on every possible tangent, even though there are many. In the context of HCTDs, it is particularly important to choose our thread and follow it, especially when working with patients who have tried absolutely everything and are genuinely worn out by their efforts. We have many schools of thought from which to choose, but choose we must.

5   In 2017, the Food and Drug Administration (FDA) delivered a clear warning of the danger posed by these antibiotics and specifically named people living with Marfan syndrome and Ehlers-Danlos syndrome as being vulnerable: "FDA warns about increased risk of ruptures or tears in the aorta blood vessel with fluoroquinolone antibiotics in certain patients" (tinyurl.com/bdeukp5j). A 2021 report by Sankar *et al.*, "Association of fluoroquinolone prescribing rates with black box warnings from the US Food and Drug Administration," investigated decreasing rates of fluoroquinolone prescription as a result of FDA warnings and noted that, "Fluoroquinolones are not the recommended first-line therapy for sinusitis and uncomplicated UTIs, yet they are among the top 4 most commonly prescribed antibiotic classes." According to their study, PCPs continue to prescribe these antibiotics despite FDA communications, while clinicians at teaching hospitals reduced their rate of prescription as a result of the newer black box warnings (tinyurl.com/2rrnjy2x). A 2022 article by Tate, "Doctors still overprescribing fluoroquinolones despite risks," references Sankar *et al.*, outlines the plight of two women who were profoundly damaged by these antibiotics, and compares the American system of black box antibiotic delivery with Australia's safer methods (tinyurl.com/7wedha72). The patient visit took place before the 2018 CDC change in warning and I was more circumspect back then. If I were confronted with a patient situation like that today, I would simply pull up the CDC statement and print it out for the person. Patients need to know this information.

6   In my practice, I educate patients regarding the benefits of Chinese medicine's approach to diet but do not prescribe dietary regimens in accordance with scope-of-practice law in Texas. I am also a certified health coach

with a specialty certification in sports nutrition, and this is helpful from a comparative perspective. Patients understand Chinese dietetics better when I can refer to common received wisdom regarding diet and then compare it with Chinese approaches. The certification also allows me to educate but not prescribe in order to remain within scope of practice. Each practitioner can check their local laws for guidance regarding this matter. Whether or not a practitioner feels like acquiring extra certifications, it is still a good idea to become familiar with what the biomedical side has to say about nutrition and HCTDs. A somewhat dated but good article about supplements is Mantle, Wilkins and Preedy's "Nutritional, therapeutic strategy for Ehlers-Danlos syndrome" (tinyurl.com/5easffju).

7   *Chinese Medicine Dietetics Volume I* (Pang and White 2014) and *Chinese Medicine Dietetic Remedies* (Pang and White 2011) can be useful for patient education. These are short books with simple, clear guidelines, and a patient can easily use them as desk references.

8   Olson *et al.* analyzed the connection between fat shaming and physical pain in "The pain of weight-related stigma among women with overweight or obesity," and found that there is a correlation between the two (tinyurl. com/yzb2y4dm).

9   Weight, body image, and a desire for some measure of control over a body that may feel like a betrayer can also precipitate eating disorders. This 2021 case study, "A young woman with excessive fat in lower extremities develops disordered eating and is subsequently diagnosed with anorexia nervosa, lipedema, and hypermobile Ehlers-Danlos syndrome" (Wright and Herbst), is instructive. Though the authors center on lipedema and self-esteem, my focus immediately went to the EDS diagnosis (tinyurl. com/yc6m3djn). Either way, the overall narrative surrounding the patient is consistent with what I have seen in my clinic with patients who have both an HCTD and issues with their weight or size. By simply being kind, respectful, and a source for healthy nutrition information, we are able to support meaningful and affirming change in our hEDS patients.

10   Not all of my patients have been gravely ill but I have had to learn how to speak to patients about getting screened for lifelong chronic illnesses and I have, of course, supported patients as they become accustomed to a diagnosis that changed their lives. Palliative care organizations have excellent resources for learning how to initiate difficult topics and they tend to be culturally sensitive. The Conversation Project, for example, shares a wealth of information regarding end of life at "Conversation starter guide—additional resources" (tinyurl.com/2a6su727) and these are translated into multiple languages. It can be useful to look at these guides and see how they model ways to engage in challenging conversations. When we work with people who live with chronic illness and pain, we serve them (and ourselves) best when we mindfully practice our communication skills and

we maintain a referral list for patients who need the support of a licensed psychotherapist who specializes in chronic illness.

11  In "Misdiagnosis of Autonomic Dysfunction in EDS as Psychiatric Disorders" (in Jovin 2020, pp.600–607) internist Alan G. Pocinki, MD, begins by reminding that, "Some disorders of the autonomic nervous system, which are common in EDS patients, present with symptoms that are similar to those of certain psychiatric disorders" (p.601). This chapter, part of a resource I discuss in chapter six of *Chinese Medicine*, is followed by "Navigating Psychiatric Misdiagnosis" (pp.608–613) by psychiatrist Richard Barnum, MD. In the first, Pocinki discusses lack of sleep, hyperarousal, and extreme reactivity as an issue of autonomic nervous system dysfunction rather than trauma; in the second, Barnum illuminates the pitfalls of incorrect biomedical diagnosis of patients who are categorized as having mental health problems when, in reality, the root cause is a misfiring autonomic nervous system. A practitioner who treats EDS patients and wishes to begin via the shen will most certainly wish to read these resources and be mindful of symptom overlap.

12  Current research notes symptom overlap, a prevalence of autism and other neurodivergence in people with HCTD, and genetic connections between autism and hEDS/HSD. Casanova *et al.* argue for this theory in "The relationship between autism and Ehlers-Danlos syndromes/hypermobility spectrum disorders." According to these researchers, their "data highlight the potential relatedness of these two conditions and suggest that EDS/HSD may represent a subtype of autism" (tinyurl.com/3ekbffj3). Some of our patients will be neurodivergent, and if we have many of them, it is useful to understand that there are cultural shifts occurring in their communities. Without knowing much about the topic, a practitioner might wish to do some extra research and can easily find the organization Autism Speaks. It may be edifying to consider a detailed response to this organization, compiled by Schultz: "A roundup of posts against Autism Speaks" (tinyurl. com/2nnzkx4s). I have had a small number of neurodivergent hEDS patients and, though it is not my forte, I think that anyone who is expert in scalp acupuncture and is interested in neuro-acupuncture could find an excellent patient base in these populations. It might be a niche practice, but it could be an extremely successful and worthy endeavor.

13  Paul Unschuld includes an outline of the earliest manifestations of this syndrome, though in *Medicine in China: A History of Ideas*, he uses the term "ku." In Unschuld's interpretation, "The ku, a worm spirit, deserves special attention because it is a possible example of how the universal encounter of a region or epoch with actual parasite infestation, transformed by demonological concept and the influence of social experiences, developed into an explanatory model that was able to convince both the educated and uneducated for many centuries" (2010, p.46). I find no clinical value in his historical account, though it is interesting when compared with the description by

García, Sierra and Balám in *Wind in the Blood: Mayan Healing and Chinese Medicine* of sickness caused to children by the evil eye (1999, pp.234–239).

14   HCTDs, per se, are not Gu syndrome. However, and especially if there is post-Lyme or toxic mold involved, the herbal approaches employed by both Drs. Zhang of *Lyme Disease and Modern Chinese Medicine: An Alternative Treatment Strategy Developed by Zhang's Clinic* (2015) and several points that Dr. Fruehauf makes in his argument (he, too, offers a comprehensive herbal program) do correspond, especially if the patient presents with the addition of emotional disorder and gut health issues.

15   In the United States the FDA has begun to maintain a page that lists drugs known to have an effect on certain genotypes: "Table of pharmacogenetic associations" (tinyurl.com/yckt4rdp).

16   Awareness of the way people with HCTDs react to dental anesthesia has increased and Schubart *et al.*'s study, "Resistance to local anesthesia in people with the Ehlers-Danlos Syndromes presenting for dental surgery," analyzes data surrounding this concern (tinyurl.com/mscsmf59). A clinical trial to address unreliable reaction to numbing medications ("Local anesthetic response in Ehlers-Danlos syndrome (EDS) and healthy volunteers") is in progress, with results expected in 2025. Pharmacogenomics, or PGx, takes into account the individual's genetic predisposition to drug reactivity and is an option for people with hEDS. See Kekic's "Medication genetics and EDS" (tinyurl.com/a8a6y8rr). It has been suggested to me that I participate in two ongoing research trials but I have thus far resisted.

17   Aside from the issue of vascular disorder, people with EDS also tend towards blood abnormalities, as Artoni *et al.*'s study, "Hemostatic abnormalities in patients with Ehlers-Danlos syndrome" (tinyurl.com/56c4xxa8), demonstrates. This is something to keep in mind before prescribing Blood-nourishing or moving herbs.

18   See Mayo Clinic, "Hydroxyzine (oral route)" (tinyurl.com/4h6w8fkn), and Chang, "Hydroxyzine (Vistaril) for anxiety: How it works, side effects, and dosage" (tinyurl.com/24kyp357).

19   The article (tinyurl.com/45nynfk6) is also useful in that it describes overactive mast cells and their response to Chinese herbal medicine, so for a practitioner's own use, I do suggest reading it alongside the resources I outline in chapter six.


# **Chapter 4**

1   Antonio Machado (1875–1939) was a beloved Spanish poet and an important member of the Generación del '98, an artistic movement dedicated to renewal and associated with Modernism. Machado was particularly known for his poetry inspired by the countryside, his love for his wife, and the

small details of humble existence which he captured in his haiku-like poetry collected in the volume *Proverbios y Cantares*.

2   Mei Zhan's *Other-Worldly: Making Chinese Medicine through Transnational Frames* traces TCM as a concept and practice via her fieldwork in both China and the United States. One thing we learn (or perhaps it only confirms our suspicions) is that herbalism is privileged over acupuncture in China and it is not surprising to read that traditionally the hierarchy was gendered in favor of male authority in the herbal realm. However, Zhan writes, "Today the gender asymmetry between male herbalists and female acupuncturists is no longer so clear, although a number of acupuncturists in Shanghai have told me that their profession is seen as inferior to herbal medicine because they work with their hands" (2009, p.124). In a specific anecdote, one of her informants clarifies the relative value of herbalism as opposed to acupuncture and tui na. To wit: "Dr. Huang, for example, told me that at the Shanghai College of Traditional Chinese medicine (SCTCM), from which she graduated in 1962, the major in acupuncture and tuina (therapeutic massage) was nicknamed zhentuiban. When pronounced in Shanghai dialect, zhentuiban is shorthand for 'class of acupuncture and tuina' but also means 'rather below par'" (*ibid.*). I confess that reading this made me feel sad but also indignant and apparently, I am not alone in these sentiments. In his introductory remarks to *Treatment of Soft Tissue Injury with Traditional Chinese and Western Medicine*, one Feng Tian-you stoutly defended this modality. "The part dealing with the treatment of soft tissue injury is accomplished," he tartly informs, "as the result of our overcoming the incorrect idea of belittling and discriminating against traditional Chinese medicine and of the devoted study of the common and frequent diseases of the laboring people, such as pain of the neck, shoulder, arm, the lumbar region, and the leg" (1983, p.1). Though Dr. Feng's righteous ire seems more in defense of social class than of modality, I found it touching. Working with one's hands is not just a matter of pushing and pressing. Tui na is not lesser. One does not develop exceptional listening hands by being mindless or coarse. To be able to see and hear with one's fingertips is an art just as subtle as that which produces classical herbal virtuosity. When we heal with our hands, we honor Chinese medical tradition and we change lives.

3   In this regard, Lockshin's *Prince* is instructive. In his introduction, he promises to address, "how patients, doctors, and administrative systems respond to uncertainty of diagnosis" and to press against the outlines of this state of not-knowing, asking, "When doctors disagree about basic facts, is that error or is it uncertainty?" Lockshin had a very long career and his observations regarding medical uncertainty are telling. To wit: "When even experienced doctors have such startling differences of opinion, how can we claim certainty? How can we say to a patient, 'Here is what you *must*

do'? Disagreement among physicians is well known to patients who have a chronic disease, as it is to their doctors. It is not so well known to the public at large" (2017, p.66); further, he declares that, "Doctors rarely talk in public about physician disagreement—except to say (often in a court of law) that someone else is wrong. We rarely discuss the reasons we disagree: The science is uncertain. The disease is not following the textbook's rules. At the moment, we don't really know" (*ibid.*, pp.67–68). Genetic research gives us a way of knowing, true, but the thread of uncertainty will, I think, persist. I do not expect that a magic pharmaceutical drug will fix a body with disordered connective tissue. There are larger forces at work here, including but not limited to environmental injury. This is not a matter of one gene, one resolution (and biomedicine practitioners know this too).

4 Received wisdom about how Chinese physicians viewed the body runs deep but we may also refer to Karchmer's assertions in *Prescriptions for Virtuosity*. Interpretation of history does shift with time, and Karchmer notes that, "New historical research by Yi-Li Wu has already helped to demonstrate that late Imperial healers closely examined the structures of the body, even if China lacked the tradition of dissection found in Europe" (2022, p.71). Political winds of change also rewrite narratives, as he elucidates: "Like Nathan Sivin and Manfred Porkert, most contemporary doctors assert that the bodies of Western medicine and Chinese medicine are radically different. But the belief that Chinese medicine describes a functional body and Western medicine a structural body only emerged in the Communist era. During the Republican era, doctors claimed that the bodies of the two medical systems were roughly analogous" (*ibid.*, p.80).

5 I confess that I am not so virtuous a scholar that I spent much time with *Yí Lín Gaí Cuo (Correcting the Errors in the Forest of Medicine)*. I came across the translation and read it because I wanted to follow the thread of reading as much as I could find on the subject of the physical, tangible, pragmatic body in Chinese medical history. This is not a thrilling tome but I appreciate that someone (in this case Yuhsin Chung, Herman Oving, and Simon Becker 2007) cared enough to render an English-language version of it. I found it useful to follow a line of historical threads too. Hilary Smith's *Forgotten Disease: Illnesses Transformed in Chinese Medicine* (2017) traces the subject of "foot qi" from its earliest manifestations as swelling and pain in the foot and lower limb to its later iteration as beriberi to its current use to depict athlete's foot. When we would wish to contextualize the body within an overarching picture of Chinese medical history, we might choose to begin with resources like *The Making of Modern Chinese Medicine, 1850–1960* (Andrews 2014), *Neither Donkey nor Horse: Medicine in the Struggle over China's Modernity* (Lei 2014), and *Know Your Remedies: Pharmacy and Culture in Early Modern China* (Bian 2020). The historians are valuable resources for us, I think, and the aforementioned are a useful place to

start our investigation into lived practices. Though we can appreciate investigations into the scholarly traditions of the body in Chinese medical history, it behooves us to push along past them in search of more pragmatic depictions.

6   Dr. Beighton and his wife, Greta, compiled histories of syndromes and the people for whom they are named. Both *The Man Behind the Syndrome* (1986) and *The Person Behind the Syndrome* (1996) are meticulously researched and well worth reading. Peter Beighton, to be quite frank, must have been a real firecracker in his day and his utter joy (clearly shared with his wife, Greta, a nurse and researcher) in writing up stories about medical colleagues is palpable. As they share in the preface to *The Person Behind the Syndrome*, "We derived enormous enjoyment and satisfaction from that endeavor [i.e., compiling the biographies], together with considerable insight into human nature," and, as a reader, I found this comment vividly indicative of what I would find as I read their collection. Dr. and Mrs. Beighton concluded this preface with a jolly admonition to readers, "For those who aspire to eponymous immortality, the trick is to identify a 'new' syndrome and then to use an extremely cumbersome descriptive title in the initial report. If co-authorship can be avoided, so much the better. A single eponym, particular if it is harmonious or curious, will stand a better chance of being perpetuated in further publications than a long obscure title!" (*ibid.*). As a practitioner who works with mystery patients, I sincerely enjoyed being able to read vivid biographical sketches that brought syndromes both rare and common alive for me. These two books are fantastic resources for anyone who would like to learn about complex genetic illnesses in a fun way.

7   In the introduction to *Classical Chinese Medicine*, Fruehauf presents a chart setting classical perspective alongside TCM views. His comparison between how each perspective sees the body is instructive. Classical Chinese medicine, "views body as field (traditional *zang-xiang* theory: *zang-fu* are primarily viewed as functional systems)" while TCM, "views body as material entity (influence of modern anatomy: *zang-fu* are primarily viewed as structural organs)" (Liu 2019, p.xli). For critical thinking, and especially if I need to extend my thread, as it were, I compare the two modes of thought and make use of what is the more appropriate reading for the patient. In this chapter, I strive to be as open as possible to either option. Once a practitioner has become familiar with an HCTD lens, they are able to work within the school of thought that is most applicable to their training, interest, and patient needs.

8   Time and repetition and experience with different patient presentations are what build our knowledge when working with complex patients. My copy of Deadman *et al.*'s *A Manual of Acupuncture* (2007) is falling apart at the seams because I have read and reread it so often. I compare what I learn by reading case study collections with my clinical experience and

then go back yet again to Deadman *et al.* The five-volume *Pathomechanisms* series by Yán Shí-Lín and translated by Sabine Wilms (2006–2012) and the two-volume *Chinese Medicine Theories of Modern Practice* by Wiseman and Wilms (2020) are instructive, albeit somewhat dry, and very useful as a desk reference. But it is never a matter of reading one source or relying on simply that. Instead, we read broadly and widely before coming back to specifics only to expand once again. Each reading of any given section from Deadman *et al.* then becomes richer and more valuable as we choose our points and develop our strategies. A more recent point prescription text is David Hartmann's *The Principles and Practical Application of Acupuncture Point Combinations.* I would have loved this resource while still in my program because its author writes with such an accessible and cheerful tone and it is still useful to me now, even as a relatively seasoned practitioner.

9   In 2018, scientists proudly announced the discovery of a new organ, the interstitium. This is the body's network of interspaces made up of collagen fibers and fluid-filled areas beneath the skin and surrounding the gut, muscles, and blood vessels. Reactions to this discovery have been mixed. While news media touted it widely, respondents to the online open-access journal article by Benias *et al.*, titled "Structure and distribution of an unrecognized interstitium in human tissues" (tinyurl.com/fpxrreyv), garnered pushback from commentators who argued that these structures were well-known by holistic therapists and other scientific researchers. For his part, Tom Myers, the founder of Anatomy Trains, issued a commentary ("Interstitium: A statement from Tom Myers" tinyurl.com/2p87dbdp). In it, his comment, "Yay for scientists for 'discovering' this, and for linking it to cancer metastasis and showing its importance in maintaining membranes. 'Yay for us' for having understood the importance of this system (albeit its mechanical, not so much physiological) importance for the last 25 years," sums up what I view as a perfectly reasonable response. Interest in the interstitium and what it represents has given way to focus on and awareness of fascia, which I consider at the end of this chapter.

10   A finely tuned debate regarding the precise nature of the San Jiao is beyond the scope of this book. Avijgan and Avijgan's "Meraque or Triple Energizer (San Jiao): Actual or virtual organ in Traditional Medicine—A hypothetical viewpoint" (tinyurl.com/4csdp4y7) is instructive. This article started as an essay read at the 2nd International Conference on Traditional and Alternative Medicine, Beijing, 2014, and the resulting paper is an expansion of the argument for similarities between traditional Persian concepts and ancient Chinese ideas regarding hollow organs ultimately designated the Meraque in the former and the San Jiao or triple burner in the latter. Avijgan and Avijgan set forth theories beginning with conception and fetal development. In summary, "During embryonic development and after gastrulation, three

layers called the ectoderm, mesoderm and endoderm are formed. The mesoderm is the source of most of the internal organs, dividing into two layers, the somatic and the visceral, with an invisible space in between that is called the coelom. This space could possibly be the same as the Meraque/Triple Energizer/San Jiao (as a hollow organ) and, furthermore, the same as a cavitary tissue forming a pathway to connect the internal organs of the body with the surface of the body." It is interesting to learn about ancient Persian medicine from this article and, especially for someone who prefers a scientific approach to the history of medicine, insightful. For a summary of classical references to the connection of the San Jiao with the interspace between skin and muscle, or cou li, we might refer to Qu's "Structure and distribution of the San Jiao and Cou Li—Recognized interstitium in human tissues" (tinyurl.com/29h4ev3y).

11  I have not yet had a patient with Eagle syndrome but I have seen people in online communities who broach the topic of being diagnosed with it. "Bilateral carotid artery dissection due to Eagle syndrome in a patient with vascular Ehlers-Danlos syndrome: A case report" (Ikenouchi *et al.*, tinyurl.com/3kfffnx5) describes a Japanese patient with diagnosed vEDS and bilateral elongated styloid processes (aka Eagle syndrome). The patient suffered arterial dissection, which is not unheard of with vEDS, but in this instance, the vEDS diagnosis caused the Eagle syndrome to be overlooked. This is an interesting case for several reasons, but for our purposes, it is a reminder to be careful with a patient's neck and provides evidence that biomedicine misses things too. Even with the best diagnostic technology and an array of highly skilled biomedical specialists, people with EDS can be misdiagnosed or have faulty or incomplete diagnoses. This is a complicated disorder. A Chinese medicine practitioner who treats vEDS patients would probably do so under the auspices of an East–West hospital program.

12  If a patient has one relatively exceptionally tight area it can be wise to release the tension in stages. If the cause of the contracted muscle is that this is the body's one (overly) stable joint, doing too much to change that at once can rebound and the joint can then become far looser than is beneficial for the patient.

13  GB-8, baichongwo Extra point, and Yin Qiao formula can be a wonderful base strategy for MCAS patients.

14  While on the subject of qi and Blood, it is never amiss to keep in mind the vascular component with EDS. Though they do not specify which subtype of EDS that they studied, Artoni *et al.*, report in "Hemostatic abnormalities in patients with Ehlers-Danlos syndrome" that over half the cohort they investigated had bleeding disorders (tinyurl.com/56c4xxa8). In the same way we avoid "boosting the qi" or "strengthening the immune system" with autoimmune patients who already have overly active immune reactions, we will tread lightly when it comes to nourishing or moving Blood when

treating people with HCTDs, especially if the degree of vascular involvement has not been entirely ascertained.

15 The Stecco family is fascinating. Luigi Stecco is an Italian physiologist who has produced a number of excellent resources pertaining to his work, which he calls the Fascial Manipulation (FM) method. Stecco, Stecco, and Stecco's *Acupuncture Western Medicine Fascial Manipulation* (2020) outlines both fascial planes and acupuncture meridians in a side-by-side comparison. There are many reasons to appreciate il Signor Stecco, and I especially do because he is adamant in his respect for Chinese medicine. This is not someone who perpetuates an East–West interaction that privileges West over East. He repeatedly declares that his successes stem from what he knows via Asian medicine, and that, "the greatest input to the development of FM is due to acupuncture" (*ibid.*, p.ix). He also has the support of Giorgio di Concetto, the founder of the Italian School of Chinese Medicine in Bologna. His daughter, Carla, whose name we see on the cover of *Fascia*, is a noted orthopedic doctor in Padua. His son, Antonio, is in the United States, where he holds a position as a research assistant professor in the Department of Rehabilitation Medicine at NYU Grossman School of Medicine. The whole family's contribution to knowledge in the realms of fascia and Chinese medicine is stellar.

# Chapter 5

1 The McGill Pain Questionnaire was created by Canadian psychologist Ronald Melzack, a founding member of the International Association for the Study of Pain, who also developed the so-called Gate Theory of Pain with colleague Patrick Wall. Though now not as influential as it was during its heyday, the Gate Theory posited the ways that nerve pain was "gated" or modulated by the nervous system. His article discussing how he developed the McGill Questionnaire (Melzack and Raja, "The McGill Pain Questionnaire: From description to measurement") is worth reading, if only to understand how pain studies developed and flourished during the 1970s (tinyurl.com/42n6u32c), thus paving the way for how pain is contextualized even now. A follow-up essay, Mendell's "Constructing and deconstructing the Gate Theory of Pain," is also useful in this regard, because the author places the model within the context of its initial reception as a seminal theory and traces the developments of arguments both pro and con about the theory's worth (tinyurl.com/y573tacp). I'm not convinced that a practitioner of Chinese medicine needs to memorize the McGill Pain Questionnaire but, when we work with chronic pain patients, it is useful to know the history of theories regarding pain.

2 It should come as no surprise to find that EDS patients feel better when allowed to make their own choices. Though there are not many studies of

wellbeing interventions in this patient population, Kalisch *et al.*, in "Feeling good despite EDS: The effects of a 5-week online positive psychology programme for Ehlers–Danlos-Syndromes patients," found that the group allowed to select their own positive psychology intervention (PPI) derived greater benefit than the group that was assigned a PPI (tinyurl.com/2nd 3vb9wn). Though this was a small study, its findings underscore the value of allowing people to assume control over their self-care strategies.

3    Karchmer's excellent study focuses on the erosion of confidence in Chinese medicine as experienced by doctors in China. We, in other countries, have our own job to do when it comes to building our levels of confidence when speaking with patients or healthcare providers in other medical traditions. The eternal question is, of course, as Karchmer notes, "Does it work?" He points out that, "Western medicine therapies are widely assumed to work, even if many specific therapies fail or work imperfectly" (2022, p.33). He further elucidates, reminding that, "If one were pressed to explain this belief in the efficacy of Western medicine, then one might point to a vast body of research, based on randomized control trials. This form of epistemological authority, however, is a relatively recent invention that only dates to the 1950s. Joseph Dumit has argued that clinical trials are profoundly shaped by the commercial imperatives of the pharmaceutical companies that run them and are far from transparent, unambiguous arbiters of therapeutic efficacy" (*ibid.*).

4    It is unusual but patients can have an allergic reaction to acupuncture needles and I have seen two different online conversations about having extreme responses to needles. For extraordinarily sensitive patients who do want to try acupuncture, the best bet might be to try Japanese techniques that do not entail insertion of a needle; otherwise, it might be worth beginning with ear seeds or variations on acupressure.

5    HCTDs present on a spectrum and not all patients are volatile at all times. Hormone shifts in women as they go through their menstrual cycle can affect reactivity; fluctuations in stress levels, weather change, degree of fatigue, and whether or not MCAS is a factor can all influence how reactive a patient is to stimuli.

6    With some patients, I palpate and then say, "I'm thinking needles for your arms and ear seeds for your legs" (or whatever region is appropriate) and I give the patient the option to agree or to voice another preference. Other patients will tell me that today their arms hurt and they want seeds on their arm points (or wherever they do not want needles during that treatment). I firmly believe that this exchange offers a great lesson for patients. When they have options and can say that they want one or the other modality, this is an interaction that celebrates their ability to perceive their own bodies and to take part in the regulation of their own pain.

7  LR is associated with lupus and Sjögren's syndrome, while a patient with rheumatoid arthritis could be presenting with rheumatoid vasculitis. Generally, a patient in these cases will have been assessed by their MD.

8  There are a number of books that breathlessly promise that red LED therapy is magical and the answer to all problems. These may have their uses but they do not do much for a practitioner who would like to acquire professional knowledge. Good desk references are Hamblin *et al.*'s *Low-Level Light Therapy: Photobiomodulation* (2018) and Turchin's *Light and Laser Therapy: Clinical Procedures* (2017).

9  In chapter six I share resources for further study. Before even considering adding nutritional education or support to patients with MCAS, one will thoroughly study the pertinent recommended resources. MCAS is complicated and volatile, and we usually only work with the relatively moderate cases of it; as one sees by reading Dr. Afrin, the extreme cases generally are treated by a biomedical team of practitioners.

10  This is another area where a knowledgeable practitioner could build a niche practice. Like Jeannie Di Bon, below, practitioners who are skilled at tai chi or qi gong and who have the resources to build an online community could provide a valuable service to people with HCTDs. There are better resources outside of the United States than within this country, I have found. One source for EDS-aware movement therapy, Earth Balance Tai Chi, is based in the UK, for instance (https://earthbalance-taichi.com).

11  People who are interested in yoga do have online resources. For example, Jeannie Di Bon is a British movement-based therapist who is active with EDS organizations and her Zebra Club app is well regarded in the community. Her website has resources for practitioners who want to learn how to provide hEDS-safe yoga or movement sessions to patients (https://jeanniedibon.com). She also has a book, *Hypermobility Without Tears: Moving Pain-Free with Hypermobility and Ehlers-Danlos Syndrome* (2019). Another reader-friendly, informative resource is Pereira and Bridges' *Too Flexible to Feel Good: A Practical Roadmap to Managing Hypermobility* (2021).

12  My training to become a Hatha yoga instructor was a 200-hour program, which is standard for yoga teachers in the United States and quite sufficient to be able to deliver healthy, safe yoga classes to the general public. To become an Iyengar teacher at the most basic level requires a minimum of three years of study and a number of tests and assessments, as one can see at Iyengar Yoga (tinyurl.com/p9kfsxu8). On a personal level, I worked for two years with an Iyengar teacher, both in private and in her group lessons, and the body awareness I got from her instruction has stayed with me for twenty years after the last class I took with her. If a patient is interested in yoga, I think that either an Iyengar teacher or a teacher with specialized knowledge is safest for them.

13 I have not had any patients who have worked with them but www. cirquephysio.com has a good reputation within hEDS circles. They offer online services, and if I had an athletic patient who needed physical therapy, I would reach out to them to discuss a referral. Circus medicine PTs have a lot to offer our HCTD patients. As much as I have spoken about pain and HCTD over the course of *Chinese Medicine*, I would also like to point out that there are people who are able to use their bodies in a joyful way, and one such person is Scarlet Checkers, a vivacious and successful contortionist (www.scarletcheckers.com/bio).

14 I have seen mixed reviews of the Muldowney Protocol but my experience is that his approach can be helpful for a patient who is willing to go slowly. He also has a clinic on the East Coast of the United States (www.muldowneypt. com). I know of other, more vigorous, trainers and programs but since I do not know them personally and I do not have patients who have made use of their services, I am reluctant to include them here. Ultimately, I hold that we do not need to do everything and that it is useful to have trusted, known referral resources.

15 An internet search with the keywords "cosmetic acupuncture and [fill in the blank with a country name]" is instructive. Chinese medicine for beauty is worldwide and popular.

16 My preferences for skincare run to Emily Skin Soothers, a line developed by an acupuncturist father whose daughter suffered from terrible rashes as a newborn. Their "testimonials" page includes photographs of babies with severe rashes who were helped considerably by using these products (www.emilyskinsoothers.com). Another acupuncturist-created and more lux product is Joy Moy (https://joymoy.com); these are organic skincare products made in small batches by a practitioner who is obsessive about the topic of hyper-reactivity and safety. My preference is always to go with acupuncturists' products when I can, but the key point is that we know our sources and we patch test *everything* before using it on a sensitive HCTD or MCAS face.

17 There is a caveat. In my estimation, and I will reiterate: it is wise to tread lightly when it comes to the psyche of patients with chronic, lifelong illness and/or medical PTSD. Myself, I do have referral sources and I will expect that a patient works with a psychotherapist if their trauma is profound or they need more from me than my scope of practice and/ or ethics will permit. This is a consideration we must all make when we work with HCTDs. That does not mean that I do not address trauma, grief, pain, fear, or shame on my treatment table. What it does mean is that I am aware of my limits and cognizant of what my patients might need beyond them. I can help patients locate where they hold trauma within their bodies and even to a degree ameliorate its effect on, say, Liver or Lungs, but when it comes to making meaning of it? That they will safely do

with their licensed psychotherapist who is trained to work with chronic illness patients.

18  My certification is from ACE, which has a well-respected health-coaching program that is reasonably priced, especially since I maintain my personal-trainer certificate with them concurrently. Some programs are expensive and labor intensive and probably not worth the effort for someone who has already spent considerable time, energy, and money to become a licensed practitioner of Chinese medicine. Especially if the practitioner has an exercise background, ACE is more than sufficient. For an outline of the top ten programs (ACE came in at number five), view Blackbyrn's "Top ten best health and wellness coaching certifications" (tinyurl.com/95a3ynfx). This list does not change radically from year to year. When I became certified in 2015, I googled "Best health-coach certifications" and, though now there is a longer list of options, the same programs appeared then and now.

19  Dr. Liu is especially vociferous in his defense of Chinese medicine, which I find encouraging. Throughout the course of *Classical Chinese Medicine*, he reiterates his position in no uncertain terms. For instance, "Some believe that without experiments, laboratories, genetic research and a thorough application of the laws of physics to every aspect of its theory, Chinese medicine cannot be modernized. This is not modernization. We do not need a nod from the little white rabbits and mice in order to modernize Chinese medicine" (2019, p.307).

# Chapter 6

1  Themes surrounding translation and cultural competency are ample in Chinese medicine and to reiterate what is extant is beyond the scope of this book, though of course I have done my homework and read widely on this topic. This is an issue that characterized a good portion of my first career. As a student myself, for instance, studying Dante's *Commedia* while at the University of Bologna and under the direction of Emilio Pasquini, whose edition we used, was one thing; he did not trouble himself unduly about his foreign students and their ability with Italian. At Indiana University, Bloomington, the experience of reading Dante with Mark Musa, who translated not only the Florentine author but also Machiavelli, Boccaccio, Luigi Pirandello, and others, was quite different. Equally so was the experience of reading Cervantes at the University of Barcelona vs. doing so under the direction of Edward H. Friedman, my dissertation director at Indiana University. When I taught, either in Italian or in Spanish, the comprehension I expected from my students varied, depending on the level of the course in question and the student profile therein. Teaching language skills to students I hoped to eventually see in my literature classes was one thing;

quite another was to teach a literature class in the hope that the students would genuinely imbibe the texts and culture. This differed from pragmatic offerings, such as Spanish for Professional Use or even courses related to service learning. There are a *lot* of observations to make about Chinese language and culture in the context of Chinese medicine in countries not China but, in the interests of brevity, I have opted to show restraint and to simply allude, with this opening section of *Chinese Medicine*'s final chapter, to the topic's profound significance.

2   Courseault, J., *et al.*, "Folate-deficient hypermobility syndrome: A proposed mechanism and diagnosis" (tinyurl.com/m8matmpb).

3   An upcoming generation of current graduate students is also breaking new ground. At the University of Warwick in England, Sabeeha Malek is undertaking research that focuses on alteration in cell adhesion and cytoskeleton dynamics ("The role of cell adhesion and cytoskeleton dynamics in the pathogenesis of the Ehlers-Danlos Syndromes and hypermobility spectrum disorders" tinyurl.com/5n6seh4a). In the United States, Gensemer *et al.* summarized findings to date in "Hypermobile Ehlers-Danlos syndromes: Complex phenotypes, challenging diagnoses, and poorly understood causes" (tinyurl.com/2p8ftn4a) and the lab where she is a researcher tentatively identified a gene mutation, "MUSC researchers announce gene mutation discovery associated with EDS" (tinyurl.com/2v9muuwf).

4   Physical trauma can be a potential trigger for EDS expression. Refer to Hamonet *et al.*, "Brain injury unmasking Ehlers-Danlos syndromes after trauma: The fiber print" (tinyurl.com/4t53c2ud). In my clinical experience, I have treated patients who had no signs of EDS until they suffered either a concussion or whiplash, after which they developed disabling hypermobility and other comorbid conditions.

5   An astute reader will notice a pattern. To wit: many who dedicate considerable effort to compiling resources either live with EDS or love someone who does. There genuinely thrives a worldwide community of people who did their own research and then put together exceptional resources. A practitioner who wants to work with HCTDs needs to understand not just the medical aspect of it but also this unique cultural and community facet too.

6   A foundation of the study of connective tissue disorder is found in the work of Victor McKusick. Though the earliest editions of McKusick's *Heritable Disorders of Connective Tissue* are out of print and only interesting for a medical historian, the fifth edition (1993), edited by Victor A. McKusick's student, Peter Beighton, is worth finding and owning. I have a real soft spot for this book, maybe because it is hard to read and yet so very informative of the arc of knowledge regarding HCTDs. It is sobering to read of the breadth and scope of genetic connective tissue disorder. We see the people so profoundly affected and read the family stories. We learn about genetics and gene expression. This is not anything that we as acupuncturists might

use in a straight line from A to B to C. And yet, the story of the internal landscape couched in the language of genetics is a narrative we should know and be able to navigate, if only a little bit, when we specialize in HCTD treatment.

7   *Rheumatology* is truly a gem. We will note their thoughts on the relationship of biomedicine and acupuncture, for instance, "One of the special features of acupuncture is that it provides the practitioner, through questioning and examination, with a guiding pathogenic energetic principle, allowing the practitioner to connect all of the patient's pathological events (present and past), thereby creating a unique reality which can only lead to a customized treatment. This approach pointedly raises all the methodological issues regarding the assessment of the effects of acupuncture. Studies to test this can in no way be molded after the Western biomedical model, which is, after all, designed to evaluate drugs, not acupuncture" (Guillaume and Chieu 1996, p.139).

8   The current iterations of *Myofascial Pain and Dysfunction: The Trigger Point Manual* (Travell and Simons) are an irreplaceable resource for our readings on pain. Many of the Chinese medicine resources we know and respect cite these books; consequently, they are not only useful for treatment. A practitioner who speaks the language of Travell and Simons will be conversant in the parlance of acupuncture and Chinese medicine for pain.

9   Arthur Frank is a Canadian professor of sociology who has experienced chronic and debilitating disease, including cancer. His *The Wounded Storyteller: Bodies, Illness, and Ethics* illuminates my assertion in the above note regarding EDS communities. He states, and I concur, that, "Professionals bring their personal suffering into their work, and ill people discover forms of vocation in illness" (2013, p.xvii). I recommend this book and find it valuable but also acknowledged while reading it that it is, to a certain degree, meant for other academics. Avoiding writing in such a voice and style is hard when one is an academic. Like any decent humanities Ph.D., I am certainly capable of larding my discourse on pain with Merleau-Ponty quotes, indeed with the fervor of a Baptist preacher slinging Bible verse. I avoided doing so with the aim of providing an accessible, readable (and, one hopes, enjoyable) resource.

10  Her Facebook group is called "TCM for Allergy and Immunology" and it is easy to find by searching. It is for families of patients and there are questions to answer before being accepted. I wrote that I am an acupuncturist and wanted to be part of the group so that I could observe and learn and was accepted quickly. I do not get the sense that I would be allowed to remain in the group if I voiced opinions or gave suggestions. Her saved documents are informative and some of the posts by families are instructive. It is a small community and not the most active group on Facebook, but joining it could be useful for a pediatric specialist.

11 Case study literature in Chinese medicine is abundant. Another exceptionally useful source is *Case Studies from the Medical Records of Leading Chinese Experts* (Zhu and Wang 2011). Though I have a revolving set of case study books, there will always be one on my reading list. Reading any one of them alongside, say, Afrin's case studies, is edifying, especially when we are able to compare our readings to our clinic experiences.

12 In the preface to the *Pi Wei Lun*, translator Bob Flaws reminds that, "the theories and treatments of Li Dong-Yuan and Zhu Dan-xi are especially appropriate for chronic diseases with multi-pattern presentations, such as allergies, endocrine disorders, chronic viral disorders, immune deficiencies, autoimmune diseases, and cancers" (1993, p.vi). Given current trends in HCTD and CTD, it is my professional opinion that a new and heavily annotated version of the *Pi Wei Lun* would be a boon to our profession. Ideally, this would entail a multi-volume set consisting of both Li Dong-Yuan and Zhu Dan-xi's works. In a perfect world, the footnotes would be dense and copious and the bibliography staggering in length and breadth.

13 Like everyone else, I rely on *Shang Han Lun*, and *Essentials from the Golden Cabinet* as my primary resources for herbal knowledge. Both the Scheid, et al., *Chinese Herbal Medicine: Formulas and Strategies* (2009) and *Materia Medica* (Bensky *et al.* 2004) volumes are constantly in rotation on my reading list, as is *Qin Bo-Wei's 56 Treatment Methods: Writing Precise Prescriptions* (Wu 2011). Because I come from Spanish and a Mediterranean background, I read Amar and Lev's *Arabian Drugs in Early Medieval Mediterranean Medicine* (2016) for comparative purposes. But ultimately, for EDS and MCAS, Chinese medicine's resources truly are sufficient as long as we stick with the eternal mantra (aka *low and slow*).

14 Journalists and other professional writers who suffer from mystery diseases or autoimmune conditions are also a great resource. Moises Velasquez-Manoff's *An Epidemic of Absence: A New Way of Understanding Allergies and Autoimmune Diseases* (2012), for instance, is a chronicle of the author's attempts to find a cure for his own severe illness via worm therapy (infection with parasitic worms). It is like reading a detective story. Another resource is Donna Jackson Nakazawa's *The Autoimmune Epidemic*. Published in 2008, it too catalogues its author's rare, debilitating autoimmune condition. This book touts itself as "the first book of its kind" on the back cover and it delivers. From where we sit in the first quarter of the twenty-first century after COVID wrought global shifts, these books seem almost quaint but they certainly outline where things all began. We read them and go to our clinics only to see patients who suffer similar illnesses.

15 Ramey's narrative depicts a patient type who unselfconsciously categorizes non-biomedical interventions as "woo" and, no matter how much they may love "holistic mind-body medicine," they view anything other than biomedicine through that lens. I do understand patients like this. Even

so, my face froze into what was known, during my professor years, as The Patented Dr. Bruno Death Ray Glare of Doom when I read the author's comments regarding acupuncture and other non-biomedical approaches. To wit: "As any dabbler in alternatives can tell you, what begins as a serious endeavor can quickly devolve into all manner of woo" (Ramey 2020, p.55) and "most of the basic woo things I was doing were really helping me" (*ibid.*, p.58).

16 Discussion of Chinese medicine in the context of the cultures and histories of Asian diasporas and multi-generational immigrant communities goes well beyond the scope of this book. This is also outside of my realm of expertise even as a professor who taught on matters of intercultural competence. Ultimately, it is for Asian American and Pacific Islander (AAPI) and other hyphenated scholars and practitioners to create their narratives and it is for scholars and practitioners who are not Asian to respectfully listen. I did look at various Asian American Studies programs to see what they are teaching students about Chinese medicine and found that Stanford offers a course on the cultural development of TCM. In my estimation, there is room to build greater ties between Chinese medicine programs and AAPI course offerings and so I direct readers to the Association for Asian American Studies website: https://aaastudies.org for inspiration, should there be further interest. Zhan's *Other-Worldly: Making Chinese Medicine through Transnational Frames* (2009) is an important text in this regard, and I will add Elizabeth Hsu's *The Transmission of Chinese Medicine* (1999) to a reading list of sources that expand intercultural competencies in this realm.

17 In conjunction with other books that I have suggested is Miranda Brown's *The Art of Medicine in Early China: The Ancient and Medieval Origins of a Modern Archive* (2015). Another exceptional resource is the *Asian Medicine Journal of the International Association for the Study of Traditional Asian Medicine* edited by American scholar Pierce Salguero, which offers ongoing inquiry from an intercultural perspective (tinyurl.com/2huypnrp).

# Bibliography


Afrin, Lawrence B. *Never Bet Against Occam: Mast Cell Activation Disease and the Modern Epidemics of Chronic Illness and Medical Complexity*. Sisters Media, 2016.

Afrin, Lawrence B. "Some Cases of Hypermobile Ehlers-Danlos Syndrome May Be Rooted in Mast Cell Activation Syndrome." *American Journal of Medical Genetics*. Ser. C Seminars in Medical Genetics. 2021187C. October 2021. 466–472.

Amar, Zohar and Efraim Lev. *Arabian Drugs in Early Medieval Mediterranean Medicine*. Edinburgh University Press, 2016.

Andrews, Bridie. *The Making of Modern Chinese Medicine, 1850–1960*. University of Hawai'i Press, 2014.

Aspell, Rob. *The Practice of Tui Na: Principles, Diagnostics, and Working with the Sinew Channels*. Singing Dragon, 2019.

Bao Xiang'áo. *Raising the Dead and Returning Life: Emergency Medicine in the Qing Dynasty*. Translated by Lorraine Wilcox. The Chinese Medicine Database, 2012.

Beighton, Peter. *The Man Behind the Syndrome*. Springer, 1986. Reprinted 2011.

Beighton, Peter and Greta Beighton. *The Person Behind the Syndrome*. Springer, 1996.

Bensky, Dan *et al*. *Chinese Herbal Medicine: Materia Medica*. 3rd edition. Eastland Press, 2004.

Bian, He. *Know Your Remedies: Pharmacy and Culture in Early Modern China*. Princeton University Press, 2020.

Brown, Miranda. *The Art of Medicine in Early China: The Ancient and Medieval Origins of a Modern Archive*. 1st edition. Cambridge University Press, 2015.

Callison, Matt. *Sports Medicine Acupuncture: An Integrated Approach Combining Sports Medicine and Traditional Chinese Medicine*. AcuSport Education, 2019.

Ching, Nigel. *The Art and Practice of Diagnosis in Chinese Medicine*. Singing Dragon, 2017.

Clavey, Steven. *Fluid Physiology and Pathology in Traditional Chinese Medicine.* 3rd edition. Foreword by Dan Bensky. Eastland Press, 2020.

Daens, Stéphane and Isabelle Dubois-Brock *et al. Transforming Ehlers-Danlos Syndrome.* 1st edition, English. The GERSED, 2022.

Deadman, Peter and Mazin Al-Khafaji, with Kevin Baker. *A Manual of Acupuncture.* Journal of Chinese Medicine Publications, 2007.

Di Bon, Jeannie. *Hypermobility Without Tears: Moving Pain-Free with Hypermobility and Ehlers-Danlos Syndrome.* Foreword by Dr Leslie Russek. Jeannie Di Bon, 2019.

Dusenbery, Maya. *Doing Harm: The Truth About How Bad Medicine and Lazy Science Leave Women Dismissed, Misdiagnosed, and Sick.* Harper One reprint edition, 2019.

Ehrlich, Henry. *Food Allergies: Traditional Chinese Medicine, Western Science, and the Search for a Cure.* Third Avenue Books, 2014.

Fasano, Alessio and Susie Flaherty. *Gut Feelings: The Microbiome and Our Health.* The MIT Press, 2021.

Feng Tian-you. *Treatment of Soft Tissue Injury with Traditional Chinese and Western Medicine.* People's Medical Publishing House, 1983.

Flaws, Bob. Translator's Preface. *Treatise on the Spleen and Stomach: A Translation of the Pi Wei Lun.* Li Dong Yuan. Blue Poppy, 1993. pp.v–viii.

Frank, Arthur. *The Wounded Storyteller: Bodies, Illness, and Ethics.* 2nd edition. University of Chicago Press, 2013.

Fruehauf, Heiner. "Driving Out Demons and Snakes: Gu Syndrome, a Forgotten Clinical Approach to Chronic Parasitism." First published in *The Journal of Chinese Medicine*, May 1998. Accessed on 1/2/23 tinyurl.com/2fth8y85.

Fruehauf, Heiner, Interviewed by Erin Moreland and Bob Quinn. "Gu Syndrome: Treating Chronic Inflammatory Disease with Chinese Herbs." 2008. Accessed on 1/2/23 tinyurl.com/ep6ftah4.

Fruehauf, Heiner, Interviewed by Bob Quinn. "Lyme Disease: An In-Depth Interview with Heiner Freuhauf." 2011a. Accessed on 1/2/23 tinyurl.com/yja3psp8.

Fruehauf, Heiner. "Traditional Chinese Approaches to Gu Syndrome: Two 18th Century Examples." Excerpt from Heiner Fruehauf, *A Clinical Handbook for Chinese Herbal Medicine.* Hai Shan Press, 2011b. Accessed on 1/2/23 tinyurl.com/27hn5srn.

García, Hernán, Antonio Sierra, and Gilberto Balám. *Wind in the Blood: Mayan Healing and Chinese Medicine.* Translated by Jeff Conant. North Atlantic Books, 1999.

Guan, Ling. "Fascia and Traditional Chinese Medicine." In Schleip *et al.*, 2022. pp.618–625.

Guillaume, Gérard and Mach Chieu. *Rheumatology in Chinese Medicine.* Eastland Press, 1996.

Hamblin, Michael R., Cleber Ferraresi, Huang Ying-Ying, Lucas Freitas de Freitas, and James D. Carroll. *Low-Level Light Therapy: Photobiomodulation.* Tutorial Texts in Optical Engineering V. TT115. SPIE Press, 2018.

Hartmann, David. *The Principles and Practical Application of Acupuncture Point Combinations.* Foreword by John McDonald. Singing Dragon, 2020.

Hsu, Elizabeth. *The Transmission of Chinese Medicine.* 1st edition. Cambridge Studies in Medical Anthropology. Cambridge University Press, 1999.

Jovin, Diana, ed. *Disjointed: Navigating the Diagnosis and Management of Hypermobile Ehlers-Danlos Syndrome and Hypermobility Spectrum Disorders.* Hidden Stripes, 2020.

Karchmer, Eric I. *Prescriptions for Virtuosity: The Postcolonial Struggle of Chinese Medicine.* Fordham University Press, 2022.

Kuriyama, Shigehisa. *The Expressiveness of the Body and the Divergence of Greek and Chinese Medicine.* Zone Books, 1999.

Lei, Sean Hsiang-Lin. *Neither Donkey nor Horse: Medicine in the Struggle Over China's Modernity.* University of Chicago Press, 2014.

Li Dong-Yuan. *Treatise on the Spleen and Stomach: A Translation of the Pi Wei Lun.* Translated and annotated by Bob Flaws. Blue Poppy, 2004.

Li Xiu-Min and Henry Ehrlich. *Traditional Chinese Medicine, Western Science, and the Fight Against Allergic Disease.* World Scientific Press, 2016.

Liu Lihong. *Classical Chinese Medicine.* Edited and introduction by Heiner Fruehauf. Translated by Gabriel Weiss, Henry Buchtel, and Sabine Wilms. Chinese University Press, 2019.

Lockshin, Michael D. *The Prince at the Ruined Tower: Time, Uncertainty, and Chronic Illness.* Custom Databanks, 2017.

McKusick, Victor M. *Heritable Disorders of Connective Tissue.* 3rd edition. The CV Mosby Co., 1966.

McKusick, Victor M. *McKusick's Heritable Disorders of Connective Tissue.* 5th edition. Edited by Peter Beighton. Mosby, 1993.

Morris, David B. *The Culture of Pain.* University of California Press, 1993.

Muldowney, Kevin. *Living Life to the Fullest with Ehlers-Danlos Syndrome: A Guide for a Person Living with EDS to Achieve a Better Quality of Life.* Outskirts Press, 2015.

Nakazawa, Donna Jackson. *The Autoimmune Epidemic.* Foreword by Dr. Douglas Kerr. Touchstone, 2008.

Nathan, Neil. *Toxic: Heal Your Body from Mold Toxicity, Lyme Disease, Multiple Chemical Sensitivities, and Chronic Environmental Illness.* Victory Belt Press, 2018.

Neumann, Donald A. *Kinesiology of the Musculoskeletal System: Foundations for Rehabilitation.* 2nd edition. Elsevier, 2010.

O'Rourke, Meghan. *The Invisible Kingdom: Reimagining Chronic Illness.* Riverhead Books, 2022.

Pang, Jeffrey and Adam White. *Chinese Medicine Dietetic Remedies*. Continuing Education Online, 2014.

Pang, Jeffrey and Adam White. *Chinese Medicine Dietetics Volume I*. Continuing Education Online, 2011.

Pereira, Celest and Adell Bridges. *Too Flexible to Feel Good: A Practical Roadmap to Managing Hypermobility*. Victory Belt Publishing, 2021.

Ramey, Sarah. *The Lady's Handbook for her Mysterious Illness*. Anchor, 2020.

Ravella, Shilpa. *A Silent Fire: The Story of Inflammation, Diet and Disease*. W.W. Norton, 2022.

Saussy, Haun. *Comparative Literature in an Age of Globalization*. Annotated edition. Johns Hopkins University Press, 2006.

Scheid, Volker. *Chinese Medicine in Contemporary China: Plurality and Synthesis*. Duke University Press, 2002.

Scheid, Volker, Dan Bensky, Andrew Ellis, and Randall Barolet. *Chinese Herbal Medicine: Formulas and Strategies*. 2nd edition. Eastland Press, 2009.

Schleip, Robert, Carla Stecco, Mark Driscoll, and Peter A. Huijing. *Fascia: The Tensional Network of the Human Body: The Science and Clinical Applications in Manual and Movement Therapy*. 2nd edition. Elsevier, 2022.

Smith, Hilary A. *Forgotten Disease: Illnesses Transformed in Chinese Medicine*. Stanford University Press, 2017.

Sontag, Susan. *Illness as Metaphor*. Farrar, Straus and Giroux, 1978.

Stecco, Luigi, Carla Stecco, and Antonio Stecco. *Acupuncture Western Medicine Fascial Manipulation*. Foreword by Giorgio Di Concetto. Piccin, 2020.

Tennant, Forest. *Intractable Pain Patient's Handbook for Survival*. Tennant Foundation, 2021.

Tennant, Forest. *The Strange Medical Saga of Elvis Presley*. Tennant Foundation, 2021.

Travell, Janet G. *Myofascial Pain and Dysfunction: The Trigger Point Manual Volume 2*. Lippincott Williams & Wilkins, 1993.

Travell, Janet G. and David G. Simons. *Myofascial Pain and Dysfunction: The Trigger Point Manual*. 3rd edition. Lippincott Williams & Wilkins, 2018.

Turchin, Curtis. *Light and Laser Therapy: Clinical Procedures*. 6th edition. Curtis Turchin, 2017.

Unschuld, Paul Ulrich, trans. and annotation. *Nan-Ching: The Classic of Difficult Issues; with Commentaries by Chinese and Japanese Authors from the Third through the Twentieth Century*. University of California Press, 1986.

Unschuld, Paul Ulrich. *Medicine in China: A History of Ideas* (1985). 25th anniversary edition. University of California Press, 2010.

Unschuld, Paul Ulrich and Herman Tessenow, with Zheng Jinsheng, trans. and ed. *Huang Di Nei Jing Su Wen: An Annotated Translation of Huang Di's Inner Classic – Basic Questions: 2 volumes*. University of California Press, 2011.

Velasquez-Manoff, Moises. *An Epidemic of Absence: A New Way of Understanding Allergies and Autoimmune Diseases*. Scribner, 2012.

Walker, Amber. *Mast Cells United: A Holistic Approach to Mast Cell Activation Syndrome*. Kindle Direct Publishing, 2019.

Walker, Amber. *The Trifecta Passport: Tools for Mast Cell Activation Syndrome, Postural Orthostatic Tachycardia Syndrome and Ehlers-Danlos Syndrome*. Kindle Direct Publishing, 2021.

Wang Ju-Yi and Jason D. Robertson. *Applied Channel Theory in Chinese Medicine: Wang Ju-Yi's Lectures on Channel Therapeutics*. Eastland Press, 2008.

Wang Qing-ren. *Yí Lín Gaí Cuo (Correcting the Errors in the Forest of Medicine)*. Translation and commentary by Yuhsin Chung, Herman Oving, and Simon Becker. Blue Poppy, 2007.

Wiseman, Nigel and Feng Ye. *A Practical Dictionary of Chinese Medicine*. 2nd edition. Paradigm Publications, 1998.

Wiseman, Nigel and Sabine Wilms. *Chinese Medicine: Theories of Modern Practice, Volume I & II*. Paradigm, 2020.

Wu Bo-Ping. *Qin Bo-Wei's 56 Treatment Methods: Writing Precise Prescriptions*. Translated and edited by Jason Blalack. Eastland Press, 2011.

Xuē Jǐ. *Categorized Essentials of Repairing the Body Zhèng Ti Lèi Yào*. Translated by Lorraine Wilcox. The Chinese Medicine Database, 2017.

Yán Shí-Lín and Lǐ Zhèng-Huá. *Pathomechanisms of the Kidney Shèn Zhī Bìng Jī*. Edited by Nigel Wiseman and Anthony Venuti. Translated by Sabine Wilms. Paradigm Publications, 2012.

Yang Shou-Zhong, trans. *Extra Treatises Based on Investigation and Inquiry: A Translation of Zhu Dan-xi's Ge Zhi Yu Lun*. Blue Poppy, 2004.

Yuè Hánzhēn. *Explanations of Channels and Points Vol. I*. Translated by Michael Brown. Edited by Allen Tsaur. Purple Cloud Press, 2019.

Zeng Sheng-ping, Jake Paul Fratkin, and Wang Jing. *TCM Case Studies: Autoimmune Disease*. People's Medical Publishing House, 2014.

Zhan, Mei. *Other-Worldly: Making Chinese Medicine through Transnational Frames*. Duke University Press, 2009.

Zhang Jingyue. *Complete Compendium of Zhang Jingyue, Vol. 1-3: Eight Principles, Ten Questions, and Mingmen Theory*. Translated by Allen Tsaur. Edited by Michael Brown. Purple Cloud Press, 2020.

Zhang Qingcai and Yale Zhang. *Lyme Disease and Modern Chinese Medicine: An Alternative Treatment Strategy Developed by Zhang's Clinic*. Sino-Med Research Institute, 2015.

Zhang, Yanhua. *Transforming Emotions with Chinese Medicine: An Ethnographic Account from Contemporary China*. Annotated edition. State University of New York Press, 2007.

Zhang Zhongjing. *Shāng Hán Lùn: On Cold Damage*. Translation and commentary by Craig Mitchell, Féng Yè, and Nigel Wiseman. Paradigm Publications, 1999.

Zhang Zhongjing. *Synopsis of Prescriptions of the Golden Chamber*. Translated by Luo Xiwen. New World Press, 1987.

Zhu Bing and Wang Hongcai, eds. *Case Studies from the Medical Records of Leading Chinese Acupuncture Experts*. International Acupuncture Textbooks. Singing Dragon, 2011.

# Index

# Acknowledgments

A book is a scholar's gift to readers both current and, one hopes, future. Such an endeavor is not created in a vacuum but is, instead, the fruit of many books and teachings that came before its construction. I have a number of people to thank for this book. First and foremost, I would like to express my gratitude to my two most important teachers. Each one has provided the foundation of my knowledge in my two careers, the first as a Spanish professor and the second as a practitioner and scholar of Chinese medicine.

My dissertation director who guided me through my first graduate program and the doctorate, Professor Edward H. Friedman, molded me as a reader, a thinker, and a writer. My mentor during my second graduate program, this time in Chinese medicine rather than in Hispanic literature, taught me all that I know about tui na and acupuncture. In so doing, he opened the gates of Chinese medicine to me. Dr. Yongxin Fan is my inspiration as a clinician. The bond of teacher and student is a lifelong one that bears offspring in the form of books and works. I sincerely hope that this scholarly "grandchild" I am producing in the lineage of Dr. Friedman and Dr. Fan is a worthy demonstration of their investment in me.

The best of this book is a testament to them; any errors or omissions are a reflection of my failings.

My mother sent me off to my first graduate program with the advice to find scholars whose work I loved and to read their best essays carefully. She urged me to use them as examples for my own work and I did just this. I used to sit with my favorite theorists and hand-copy their works so that I could learn to write in my own voice but with echoes of those who came before me. My mother was a scholar in her own right, albeit in English literature rather than Spanish and Italian like me. One of my most cherished memories of my mom is that she would read the theorists whose work I loved, even though we were in different fields, just so that she could know what mattered to me as a budding intellectual. If she were with us now, I would tell her that yes, she was right about a certain critic being dry as toast. But at the time? Well. I am so grateful for her confidence in my academic abilities. And though we had our conflicts, I know that my mother would read this book and be so proud of me.

As I thank the women scholars who contributed to my development, I cannot forget the late Dr. Frances Wyers. I still have some of the books she left me, and one of her seminal essays, "El Acoso: Alejo Carpentier's War on Time," was one that I copied by hand as I learned to write as a theorist and literary critic. I am proud to know that my writer's voice shows not only the influence of Dr. Friedman's guidance but also that of Dr. Wyers. In my second career, I remain grateful to Dr. Zheng, my clinical supervisor for my Friday rotations during the final year of my program. She was so loving and kind. I don't know any student intern who didn't adore Dr. Zheng, and her example of kindness not only to interns but also to patients was a lesson to us all.

This book is a grandchild to my late mother, to Dr. Wyers, and to Dr. Zheng, too, and I offer it with my gratitude to these women in my life who have meant so much to me.

There are other significant teachers who also warrant my gratitude. Dr. Qianzhi Wu's courses on the foundations of Chinese medicine and the classics of same instilled a solid core of knowledge that I rely upon to this day. Dr. Yuxin He's series on herbal treatment of disease will stay with me forever, as will Dr. Liu's syndromes class. Dr. Xiaotian Shen generally filled my heart with terror when I was a new student but I learned so much from his classes. I hope that this book honors my teachers who came from China to Texas to share their cultural treasures with me and my fellow students. When I am successful in clinic and with this book, it is a living act of gratitude for their hard work to pass on their knowledge.

There are many people to thank for my knowledge of Chinese medicine, and I would be remiss if I neglected the resources that made my continued development possible. As I wrote this book, I began to feel like Sabine Wilms was a constant companion in this endeavor. Her translations bring a treasure house of knowledge to those of us who do not yet speak Chinese and are unable to read classical texts in the original. Resources from her publishing house, Happy Goat Productions, and other independent sources like the Purple Cloud Institute are invaluable. Eastland Press is a gem, and of all the books of theirs that I love (and I love most of them) I must single out *Applied Channel Theory in Chinese Medicine: Wang Ju-Yi's Lectures on Channel Therapeutics* (Wang and Robertson 2008) as being an inspiration and a treasure trove of learning. As a learner, I would be remiss if I did not thank Ainge Lin, whose friendship and lessons on culture, history, and language acquisition I appreciate dearly.

This book would not be possible without Singing Dragon and my editor, Claire. A thousand thank yous to Claire, and to Rosa, too, and to everyone at Singing Dragon who took part in making this volume a reality (and yes, it does take a village to create a book).

A special thank you goes to John Largess, for the many hours of discussion about books, scholarship, teaching, and wellness, and for his generosity in reading this book in draft form.

My gratitude goes to the students who taught me how to be a professor in my first career, especially those at the University of New Mexico in Albuquerque, Colorado College, and Bucknell University. I have loved my students wherever I have taught but these three are the places where I felt most at home. The process of earning my doctorate was grueling. When not studying or writing or teaching, it was training with Shaun Creighton that taught me life lessons that are with me today. I remain ever thankful for the bond that I share with Coach Shaun even now. There are people who made it possible for me to move from one career to the next and, of these guardian angels, I will forever be grateful to Steve Ravel for coming into my life at a crucial junction. I also wish to thank the patients who taught me, who trusted me, and who have shared their vulnerabilities and triumphs with me in my present iteration. When I share clinical anecdotes, it is with permission and I have altered details so that nobody will be recognizable but these are very real patients who are very dear to me. I especially wish to thank Chelsy B, who so generously took the time to read and comment on this book while it was still in manuscript form.

To my self-created family, friends, and colleagues who have remained with me during my second program, I cannot thank you enough. Heartfelt gratitude and much love goes Marlowe, Rey, Jennifer, and Kevin, especially, for their continued support and encouragement.

And to you, dear reader, I thank you for your investment in this book and for your work with hypermobile patients. You are needed and you make a difference in their lives. For people challenged by hypermobile Ehlers-Danlos syndrome, this medicine, Chinese medicine, is a gift that is worth a thousand gold coins, if not more. May you bestow it with grace and wisdom so that its benefits and blessings come back to you a hundred-fold.

Thank you.

Dr. Paula Bruno, Ph.D., L.Ac.